Principles and Practice of Sleep Telemedicine

Principles and Practice of Sleep Telemedicine

CHRISTINE WON, MD, MS

Associate Professor
Department of Medicine (Pulmonary)
Yale University School of Medicine, New Haven
Connecticut
United States
Director
Yale Sleep Center
Yale University School of Medicine, New Haven
Connecticut
United States
Director
Women's Sleep Health Program
Yale University School of Medicine, New Haven
Connecticut
United States

MEIR H. KRYGER, MD, FRCPC

Professor Emeritus
Pulmonary Critical Care and Sleep Medicine
Yale University, New Haven
Connecticut
United States

ELSEVIER

Elsevier
1600 John F. Kennedy Blvd.
Ste 1800
Philadelphia, PA 19103-2899

Content Strategist: Mary Hegeler
Senior Content Development Specialist: Shilpa Kumar
Content Development Manager: Somodatta Roy Choudhury
Publishing Services Manager: Shereen Jameel
Project Manager: Haritha Dharmarajan
Design Direction: Renee Duenow

Printed in India

Last digit is the print number: 9 8 7 6 5 4 3 2 1

Working together
to grow libraries in
developing countries

www.elsevier.com • www.bookaid.org

Dedication

To our children
Ella Chun, Sofia Chun
Shelley Gold, Michael Kryger, Steven Kryger-Even

CONTRIBUTORS

Vivian Asare, MD
Assistant Professor
Sleep Medicine
Yale University
New Haven, Connecticut

Charles Bae, MD, MHCI, FAASM
Associate CMIO for Connected Health
  Strategy
Associate Professor of Medicine
  and Neurology
Sleep Medicine
University of Pennsylvania
Philadelphia, Pennsylvania

Michelle T. Cao, DO
Clinical Professor of Medicine
Pulmonary and Critical Care Medicine
Stanford University School of Medicine
Palo Alto, California

Innessa Donskoy, MD FAAP, FAASM
Attending Physician
Pediatric Sleep Medicine
Advocate Children's Hospital
Park Ridge, Illinois

Jennifer Joan Dorsch, MD
Assistant Professor of Clinical Medicine
Sleep Medicine
University of Pennsylvania
Philadelphia, Pennsylvania

Barry Fields, MD, MSEd
Associate Professor
Division of Pulmonary, Allergy, Critical
  Care, and Sleep Medicine
Emory University, Atlanta
Georgia

Janet Hilbert, MD
Associate Professor of Clinical Medicine
Division of Pulmonary, Critical Care, and
  Sleep Medicine
Yale School of Medicine
New Haven, Connecticut

Seema Khosla, MD, FCCP, FAASM
Medical Director
Sleep
North Dakota Center for Sleep
Fargo, North Dakota

Kullatham Kongpakpaisari
Fellow
Pulmonary Critical Care and Sleep
Yale University
New Haven, Connecticut

Meir H. Kryger, MD, FRCPC
Professor Emeritus
Pulmonary Critical Care and Sleep Medicine
Yale University
New Haven, Connecticut

William F. Martin, PsyD, MPH, MSc
Professor
Department of Management &
  Entrepreneurship
DePaul University
Chicago, Illinois
Research and Innovation Leadership Fellow
Office of Research Services
DePaul University
Chicago, Illinois
Founder and CEO
Zesty Sleep, LLC
Chicago, Illinois

Anne Marie Morse, DO
Director
Child Neurology and Pediatric Sleep Medicine
Geisinger, Janet Weis Children's Hospital
Danville, Pennsylvania

Sreelatha Naik, MD
Director, Sleep Medicine; Associate,
  Pulmonary and Critical Care Medicine
Pulmonary, Critical Care and Sleep Medicine
Geisinger Health System
Wilkes-Barre, Pennsylvania

Thomas Penzel, PhD
Research Director
Interdisciplinary Sleep Medicine Center
Charité - Universitätsmedizin Berlin, Berlin
Berlin
Germany

Susan Rubman, PhD
Assistant Professor
Department of Clinical Psychiatry
Yale School of Medicine
New Haven, Connecticut
Director, Behavioral Sleep Medicine
Pulmonary/Sleep Medicine
UConn Health
Farmington, Connecticut

Ashima S. Sahni, MD
Assistant Professor of Clinical Medicine
Division of Pulmonary, Critical Care, Sleep
    and Allergy
University of Illinois at Chicago
Chicago, Illinois

Therese Santiago
Therese Santiago MA
Pre-medical Program,
Johns Hopkins University,
Krieger School for Arts and Sciences
Baltimore, Maryland

Lynelle Schneeberg, PsyD
Fellow, American Academy of Sleep Medicine
Assistant Professor of Clinical Psychiatry
Psychiatry
Yale School of Medicine
New Haven, Connecticut
Director, Pediatric Behavioral Sleep
    Medicine Program
Sleep Center
Connecticut Children's Medical Center
Farmington, Connecticut

**Sharon Schutte-Rodin, MD, DABSM, FAASM,
CBSM**
Adjunct Professor of Medicine
Sleep Medicine
University of Pennsylvania Perelman School
    of Medicine
Philadelphia, Pennsylvania

Arveity Setty, MD, FAASM, FAAP
Sleep Specialist
Pediatrics
Sanford Health
Fargo, North Dakota
Clinical Associate Professor
Pediatrics
University of North Dakota: School
    of Medicine and Health Sciences
Fargo, North Dakota
Medical Director
Sleep Center
RiverView Health, Crookston
Minnesota

Shannon Sullivan, MD
Clinical Professor
Pediatric/Sleep
Stanford University
Palo Alto, California
Clinical Sciences Team Lead
Verily Life Sciences, South
San Francisco, California
Evidenced Based Health Care, MSc Program
Nuffield Department of Primary Care
    Health Sciences
Oxford University, Oxford
United Kingdom

Srithika Thapa
Assistant Professor of Medicine (Pulmonary)
Pulmonary Critical care and Sleep Medicine
Yale University
New Haven, Connecticut

Ian Weir, DO
Program Director
Sleep Fellowship
Norwalk Hospital
Norwalk, Connecticut

Christine Won, MD, MS
Associate Professor
Department of Medicine (Pulmonary)
Director
Yale Sleep Center
Director
Women's Sleep Health Program
Yale University School of Medicine
New Haven, Connecticut

Aspects of telemedicine have been adopted in sleep medicine for decades. Home sleep testing and remote monitoring of PAP devices are just two examples. The COVID-19 pandemic has brought about a paradigm shift in the way health care in general and sleep medicine in particular are delivered. The need for social distancing and the risk for infection have led to the widespread adoption of telemedicine. Telemedicine has been widely adopted in the field of sleep medicine, which has traditionally relied on in-person consultations and in-facility sleep testing. During the COVID-19 public health emergency, The American Academy of Sleep Medicine (AASM) recommended telemedicine as a viable alternative to in-person consultations. During this dire period, telemedicine enabled sleep clinicians to provide care to patients remotely, without the need for them to visit a sleep center or laboratory. This was particularly beneficial for patients who lived in remote areas or had mobility issues.

Since the end of the COVID-19 public health emergency, the use of telemedicine in sleep medicine has continued. The benefits of telemedicine in sleep medicine are numerous. Telemedicine has made it easier for patients to access care, regardless of their location. Patients no longer have to travel long distances to visit a sleep center or laboratory.

Telemedicine has also been beneficial for sleep clinicians. It has enabled them to provide care to a larger number of patients without the need for additional staff or resources. Telemedicine has also made it easier for sleep clinicians to collaborate with other health care professionals, such as primary care physicians and specialists. This has the potential to lead to more favorable patient outcomes and improved quality of care.

This is the first book that reviews the many aspects of telemedicine that affect the clinician caring for patients who have sleep disorders. Telemedicine, once a novelty, is now an important part of clinical care and will evolve further as technology evolves.

Christine Won, MD
Meir Kryger, MD, FRCPC

ACKNOWLEDGMENTS

We thank the authors who started their chapters during the dark days of the COVID-19 pandemic and revised them as the public health emergency was lifted. We thank the staff of Elsevier (Mary Hegeler, Shilpa, and Haritha Dharmarajan) for their hard work on bringing this book to final publication.

CONTENTS

SECTION V   *Telemedicine Diagnostics and Management*

Introduction

CHAPTER 1

Introduction to Sleep Telemedicine

Christine Won ■ Meir H. Kryger

What Is Telemedicine?

The elements of telemedicine have been available for several decades. *Telemedicine* is a general term that is currently used to describe the delivery of health services that substitutes electronic systems for in-person communication between patients and health care providers; communication between providers; and patient or provider contact with information sources (e.g., medical literature, practice guidelines, algorithms, websites).[1] The term was first introduced in 1969, well before the personal computer or the Internet was developed.[2]

For the aforementioned capabilities to exist, the following historical advances were required: computer systems, mass storage, networks, the Internet, computer audio, computer video, and smart devices (phones, tablets). Telemedicine has already been implemented in other fields of medicine (e.g., diabetes and stroke).[3,4]

Other related terms are in use. *Telehealth* is usually understood to refer to the electronic systems that maintain the health of the population (e.g., epidemiology, health care systems, insurance carriers, the VA Healthcare system, CMS, clinics). *E-Health* is a neologism, vaguely defined and similar to other invented terms (e.g., *e-commerce, e-government, e-education*) introduced as use of the Internet expanded. *M-Health* is a term used to describe the use of mobile technology (smart phones, tablets, networks, portable sensors) in the delivery of health care.

As described later in this chapter, almost all elements of sleep telemedicine were already in use by 2019, and the trigger to transition to 100% telemedicine was the coronavirus disease 2019 (COVID-19) pandemic in 2020. Sleep medicine clinics had already implemented remote sleep test interpretation, interrogation of positive airway pressure (PAP) devices, and setting of PAP parameters. Once the pandemic struck, transition was necessary to protect patients and staff and to comply with Centers for Disease Control and Prevention (CDC) and state guidelines and mandates. The transition became financially sustainable with provision of new billing codes and changes in licensing so patients could be managed in locations other than their home jurisdictions.

The Dimensions of Sleep Telemedicine

There are at least three dimensions of sleep telemedicine (Figure 1.1). These are the basic functions of a clinical program, the specialized functions of the program, and the technology that enables the functions. Here we will use the term *provider* to refer to anyone involved in the management of patients, such as clinicians, front office staff, back office staff, technicians, health system administrators, pharmacists, and equipment providers.

BASIC FUNCTIONS OF A CLINICAL PROGRAM

Communication. All clinical programs rely on two-way communication between providers (e.g., consultations, referrals); between patients and providers; and between clinics and insurance

3

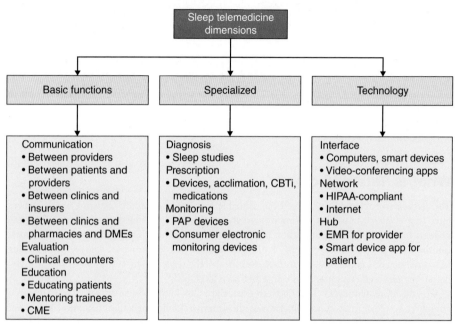

Figure 1.1 The dimensions of sleep telemedicine. Except for patient encounters, almost all aspects of sleep telemedicine were available and often used. The COVID-19 pandemic hastened the inevitable expansion of sleep telemedicine. *CBTi,* Cognitive behavioral therapy for insomnia; *CME,* Continuing medical education; *COVID-19,* coronavirus disease 2019; *DME,* durable medical equipment; *EMR,* electronic medical record; *HIPAA,* Health Insurance Portability and Accountability Act; *PAP,* positive airway pressure.

carriers. Telemedicine communication is only possible if the necessary hardware (smart phone, tablet, or computer) and electronic backbone (network) are available to all participants (see later).

Evaluation. The medical encounter between the clinician and patient is the most important act in medicine. A detailed history and physical examination are paramount, leading to a differential diagnosis, testing, and ultimately to treatment.

Education. Patient education is key to successful diagnosis and treatment. An important function of many clinical programs is to mentor the next generation. Of course, continuing education is necessary for providers to maintain skills and stay up to date in their field.

Of all of the aforementioned functions, only one—the medical encounter between the patient and provider—was generally not being performed (or could not be performed) using telemedicine. Technology (see later) was able to emulate aspects of the clinical encounter at least partially.

SPECIALIZED FUNCTIONS OF A CLINICAL SLEEP MEDICINE PROGRAM

Diagnosis. As a result of the clinical encounter between the patient and provider, diagnostic tests are ordered, including in-laboratory polysomnograms, multiple sleep latency tests (MSLTs), home sleep apnea tests, and blood tests. Systems are available to monitor in an ambulatory setting all variables collected during in-laboratory testing, except there are no ambulatory surrogates as yet for the MSLT or when in-laboratory testing is needed (e.g., split night sleep studies, titration studies, testing requiring special equipment such as transcutaneous carbon dioxide).

Prescription. After a diagnosis is made, the provider may order devices (e.g., PAP devices, mandibular advancement devices), cognitive behavioral therapy, and medications. The ordering can be done electronically. Paradoxically, communications among clinics, pharmacies, and durable medical equipment companies (DMEs) are often still via fax, a very outdated technology.

Monitoring. Systems were already available to monitor adherence and efficacy of patients being treated with PAP devices. Patients are also able to monitor how they are doing using smart devices. Besides monitoring the PAP device, many patients are using consumer technology to monitor their oxygen saturation. For the vast majority of consumer oximetry devices (fingertip, ring, wrist worn), validity is still an issue, especially for darkly pigmented people.[5-8]

TECHNOLOGY

Interface. Computers, smart devices, and video-conferencing apps have made telemedicine feasible. One can make health care available to a patient in almost any location where a network is available using two-way voice and visual communication (by computer or smart device). Many patients may have difficulty with this due to lack of smart devices or because of lack of familiarity in using computers or smart devices. Access and equity were and continue to be problematic.[9]

Network. A network is the cornerstone of communications between the provider and patient. The network could be a cellular network or the Internet. The communication must be compliant with the Health Insurance Portability and Accountability Act of 1996 (HIPAA). This may be a hurdle for some patients, or their connection to a network is poor, or the network does not have the bandwidth to allow for efficient communication.

This connects all the aforementioned functions. The electronic medical record (EMR) system is used to document and store the information of all encounters, prescriptions, treatments, and data. It is used to communicate with the patient. The patient using a smart device can access the hub and the information stored in the hub.

COVID-19 and Uptake of Sleep Telemedicine

Within days of declaration of the pandemic emergency, most sleep medicine programs were able to transition to a telemedicine model, often with the provider working from home. As mentioned earlier, most sleep medicine functions were already being performed using telemedicine. The missing piece was the ability to do the encounter with the patient. Providers set up systems in their homes (Figure 1.2). Patient were instructed on how to set up their computer or cell phone for the encounter. Both the provider and patient had to have the technical capability and the devices and networks to be able to have a successful encounter. This was often a hurdle.

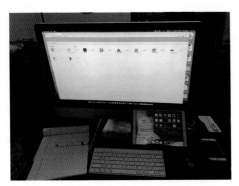

Figure 1.2 The requirements of a "home office" to successfully complete many aspects of a face-to-face encounter. Needed are a high-speed network, a computer and/or tablet, connection to a hub by a virtual private network (VPN), and video-conferencing software. A phone is needed in case the patient is unable to connect via video. Note the thermometer on the table. This was used early in the pandemic to make sure the provider did not have a fever. This was a requirement of the author's institution as part of a daily health check.

Papers per year

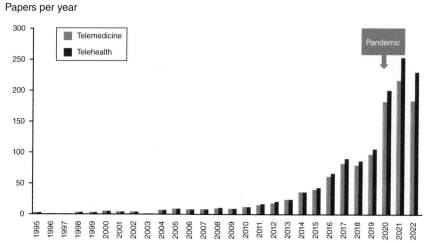

Figure 1.3   The number of publications about telemedicine and sleep mirrored the technological advancements in the past 20 years. There was a dramatic increase in publications in 2020 during the COVID-19 pandemic. *COVID-19,* Coronavirus disease 2019.

Most sleep medicine programs transitioned to using telemedicine within days to weeks. As mentioned earlier, many aspects of sleep medicine were already being performed remotely (e.g., interpretation of sleep studies, prescriptions, messaging to patient via EMR platforms). There were obviously teething pains. The number of articles about sleep and telemedicine or telehealth on PubMed skyrocketed in 2020 and 2021 (Figure 1.3).

The Future Is Now

Because telemedicine is so convenient and cost-effective for many if not most patients, many aspects are likely to continue as governments, insurers, and professional societies see the advantages.[10] It is likely that some changes in patient management (e.g., cognitive behavioral therapy for insomnia [CBTi]) are unlikely to revert to pre-COVID-19 processes.[11,12] See Chapter 4 for changes in reimbursement with telemedicine post-pandemic.

Consumer-facing devices are becoming increasingly sophisticated so one can obtain actionable data to better assess and follow patients.[13]

Despite many advantages of telemedicine, an important issue remains—health equity. Barriers on the provider side include availability of technology and personnel. Significant barriers for many patients include cost of technology, language, culture, and educational level. It is unclear whether telemedicine improves or worsens health equity.[14]

Telemedicine can be extremely convenient for patients. They do not have to take an entire morning or day off work or other activities to attend what is often a short visit. Patients may not have to travel at all. We have performed telemedicine visits with patients who were in their homes, vehicles (trucks, automobiles, boats, buses), and workplaces (factories, retail outlets). Such encounters often give the clinician an excellent picture of the patient's life. Very often, when additional information was needed from family members, one could ask the family member to pop into the encounter. Sometimes family members help facilitate the encounters.

During the pandemic, some states in the United States changed medical licensing rules and allowed practitioners from other states to see patients in their area. International telemedicine has started and is likely to expand.

Most clinics will continue to have at least some, or perhaps a great deal of telemedicine. The future is exciting.

The following chapters will outline the aspects of sleep telemedicine in granular detail. Finally, sleep medicine will be able to take advantage of the technological revolution that has affected so many aspects of our lives.

References

1. Bashshur R, Shannon G, Krupinski E, Grigsby J. The taxonomy of telemedicine. *Telemed J E Health*. 2011;17(6):484-494.
2. Murphy R, Bird K. Tele-medicine and occupational health services. In: *Proceedings of the XVI International Congress on Occupational Health*. 1969:385-387.
3. Jeong JY, Jeon JH, Bae KH, et al. Smart care based on telemonitoring and telemedicine for type 2 diabetes care: multi-center randomized controlled trial. *Telemed J E Health*. 2018;24(8):604-613.
4. Kim DK, Yoo SK, Park IC, et al. A mobile telemedicine system for remote consultation in cases of acute stroke. *J Telemed Telecare*. 2009;15(2):102-107.
5. Luks AM, Swenson ER. Pulse oximetry for monitoring patients with COVID-19 at home. Potential pitfalls and practical guidance. *Ann Am Thorac Soc*. 2020;17(9):1040-1046.
6. Modi AM, Kiourkas RD, Li J, Scott JB. Reliability of smartphone pulse oximetry in subjects at risk for hypoxemia. *Respir Care*. 2021;66(3):384-390.
7. Philip KEJ, Bennett B, Fuller S, et al. Working accuracy of pulse oximetry in COVID-19 patients stepping down from intensive care: a clinical evaluation. *BMJ Open Respir Res*. 2020;7(1):e000778.
8. Sjoding MW, Dickson RP, Iwashyna TJ, Gay SE, Valley TS. Racial bias in pulse oximetry measurement. *N Engl J Med*. 2020;383(25):2477-2478.
9. Chang JE, Lai AY, Gupta A, Nguyen AM, Berry CA, Shelley DR. Rapid transition to telehealth and the digital divide: implications for primary care access and equity in a post-COVID era. *Milbank Q*. 2021; 99(2):340-368.
10. Shamim-Uzzaman QA, Bae CJ, Ehsan Z, et al. The use of telemedicine for the diagnosis and treatment of sleep disorders: an American Academy of Sleep Medicine update. *J Clin Sleep Med*. 2021;17(5): 1103-1107.
11. Sharafkhaneh A, Salari N, Khazaie S, et al. Telemedicine and insomnia: a comprehensive systematic review and meta-analysis. *Sleep Med*. 2022;90:117-130.
12. Manber R, Alcántara C, Bei B, Morin CM, van Straten AA. Integrating technology to increase the reach of CBT-I: state of the science and challenges ahead. *Sleep*. 2023;46(1):zsac252.
13. Arroyo AC, Zawadzki MJ. The implementation of behavior change techniques in mhealth apps for sleep: systematic review. *JMIR Mhealth Uhealth*. 2022;10(4):e33527.
14. Szymczak JE, Fiks AG, Craig S, Mendez DD, Ray KN. Access to what for whom? How care delivery innovations impact health equity. *J Gen Intern Med*. 2023;38(5):1282-1287.

CHAPTER *2*

COVID-19 and Crisis-Driven Adoption of Telemedicine

Seema Khosla ■ Indira Gurubhagavatula

Background

SARS-CoV-2 changed the landscape of health care delivery abruptly and broadly,[1] resulting in a loss of access to diagnostic and therapeutic services for some patients, with preservation in others. Medical practices were challenged to recreate clinic visits and diagnostic testing in a way that emphasized strategies to mitigate transmission, including physical distancing, masking, and ventilation. Numerous strategies were instituted rapidly, including canceling or delaying non-urgent procedures, using telemedicine when possible, and triaging in-person medical care based on urgency and severity of disease by patients and by health care providers after balancing viral exposure against the need for immediate attention. As a result of care avoidance, the diagnosis and care of sleep disorders was postponed for some patients. The global impact of these choices on known health, safety, and performance outcomes of untreated or undertreated sleep disorders is unknown.

Initial guidance by the U.S. Centers for Disease Control and Prevention (CDC) to mitigate SARS-CoV-2 transmission focused on strategies to curb spread via droplets. Data continued to emerge that SARS-CoV-2 was, in fact, spread through the airborne route.[2,3] Infections among health care workers appeared to be higher among those who performed airway interventions, including otorhinolaryngologists and anesthesiologists, among others. Data that were extrapolated from Toronto during an earlier SARS-CoV-1 pandemic showed that respiratory therapists who conducted airway-stimulating procedures, such as administering nebulizers or high-flow oxygen, were at higher risk. As a result, the CDC eventually advised physical distancing and wearing face coverings to reduce airborne transmission. Furthermore, positive airway pressure (PAP) therapy is known to generate aerosols and was implicated in an early outbreak of SARS-CoV-2 in a nursing home facility in Washington state.[4,5] A total of 129 residents were infected, and 23 died in that outbreak. PAP titration studies performed in sleep laboratories were therefore designated as high-risk procedures. The risk for transmission to household members also became a concern for patients who were prescribed chronic PAP therapy for home use and lacked the ability to isolate themselves from others upon infection.

The need for clear and specific guidance was in high demand among clinicians and laypersons at a time when hard evidence was lagging. In the interim, many clinical practices sought to continue to offer medical care while developing protocols to minimize risk to patients and staff. The vast majority[6] embraced telemedicine to accomplish both of these goals. Professional societies created specialty-specific guidance based on best-available evidence to support sleep medicine practices seeking to conduct initial and return visits via telemedicine as well as guidance regarding safe treatment options.

Sleep medicine as a field implemented telemedicine[6] broadly and swiftly. Some practices were already well-versed in telemedicine technologies and had a robust infrastructure in place. Others began anew. Even clinical practices with legacy systems that were designed for center-to-center sleep telemedicine (such as the Veterans' Administration) needed to adapt to center-to-home (C2H) or home-to-home (H2H) telemedicine protocols.

In addition to clinic visits, telemedicine also required adaptation of sleep laboratory protocols. Although sleep clinicians were already very familiar with home sleep apnea testing (HSAT), these devices were usually dispensed to the patient during the course of a clinic visit. As in-person clinic visits shifted to telemedicine visits, deployment of HSAT equipment needed to be reevaluated. Many facilities developed drive-by pickup options with remote education done via teleconference, telephone, or short, pre-prepared videos. Others adopted mail delivery. Some practices used disposable HSAT devices to eliminate the risk of device loss, the need for inventory control, and the challenges of arranging for device return.

During the early period, some patients lost access to care either through lack of awareness that telemedicine visits were feasible with only a telephone or computer; lack of access to digital technology or broadband services; limited technological literacy; or lack of services. The delay or absence of care likely had a clinical impact, and a steep decrease in referrals and diagnostic testing[7] resulted in significant financial losses[6] for many individuals.

How COVID-19 Led to the Adoption of Telemedicine

If disruption can be quantified by the impact on practice change before and after said disruption, the coronavirus disease 2019 (COVID-19) pandemic was the single most significant disruptive force in the history of telemedicine. Prior to the pandemic, though some studies showed that clinicians and patients recognized the effectiveness and convenience of telemedicine, use of tele-video and/or the telephone for patient care was limited by (1) lack of sufficient reimbursement and (2) restrictions regarding eligibility, such as location in an underserved area or requirement for the clinician and patient to be located in the same state, requirement for the clinician to be in a medical facility, or requirement to have had a prior in-person visit. At the time of the pandemic, however, the Centers for Medicare and Medicaid Services (CMS) urgently passed the Telemedicine Expansion Act, which had specific clauses including parity in reimbursement for telephone or tele-video visits with in-person visits, expansion of the covered workforce, and relaxation of other previous barriers; patients and clinicians could be in any state, in any area (urban or rural), or in a non-medical facility (including a home, building, tent, or other location) during the visit. These relaxations allowed far more patients to continue to receive uninterrupted care because visits could be done with patients in their homes by using readily available audio-video technology.

Sleep medicine was uniquely positioned to adopt telemedicine at far higher rates for two reasons. First, our field relies heavily on the clinical history and physical examination components that can be assessed by tele-video. Second, the major forms of data review including sleep study testing and PAP adherence assessments were already accessible using remote access, with cloud-based, Health Insurance Portability and Accountability (HIPAA)-compliant technology. Some practices were routinely using telemedicine already and therefore demonstrated this approach to clinic visits as a viable one. Joining these practices, numerous others in the initial weeks of the pandemic efficiently evaluated and implemented new software to adapt to the C2H or H2H model. As a result of this foundational, pre-pandemic investment in technology and workflow, access to ongoing, uninterrupted care soared for many.

Nonetheless, challenges were experienced by clinicians and patients in the ensuing weeks and months because of technical reasons (insufficient bandwidth, lack of connectivity, lack of literacy with operating telemedicine software and hardware technology); physical disabilities (visual or hearing impairment, limited dexterity); and privacy and safety concerns (patients attempting visits while driving, while non-stationary, while at unsafe work locations, or in non-private locations).

In response, the American Academy of Sleep Medicine (AASM) created a telemedicine committee that published an update to a previous telemedicine position statement.[8] This expert consensus document outlined the new paradigms of sleep telemedicine to include C2H telemedicine and the utilization of patient-friendly audio-video platforms. In the early days of the pandemic, due to relaxation of regulations, these visits could be conducted via popular platforms such as FaceTime and Skype. Collaboration again was the rule, with experienced telemedicine clinicians sharing tips and tricks with less-experienced colleagues.

As time passed, clinical visits moved away from FaceTime and Skype and onto designated telemedicine platforms with enhanced features. Some of these features included a thoughtful consideration of the patient's experience. Platforms that offered one-click visits without passwords, downloads, or personal accounts proved to be the easiest from a patient standpoint. Although many patients and clinicians appreciated the convenience and efficiency, these features did not eliminate the occasional need to cancel visits due to connectivity or safety issues (e.g., patients driving). Clinicians no longer controlled both sides of the telemedicine visit. Some centers lacked administrative personnel to support, engage, and "onboard" patients before visits; instruct them about the technology; or record patient-collected vital signs or other medical data. As a result, clinicians bore the brunt of clinical as well as technological responsibilities during visits.

The AASM guidance document also advised that telemedicine visits should emulate in-person visits in content, format, and patient experience. This included history taking, data review, and performing an appropriate physical examination. Components of the examination could include positioning the patient appropriately; requesting an additional light source such as a window, lamp, or flashlight; asking patients to palpate their lower extremities to assess for edema; asking patients to open their mouth and reposition the camera to examine the oropharynx; and asking patients to turn their head to assess cranial morphology. Hands could be examined for clubbing or cyanosis. Thus, many key elements of the examination could be completed and were sufficient to allow decision-making regarding next steps; the option for in-person assessment could be reserved for those for whom such an intervention was deemed essential. Some patients had access to in-home measurement of vital signs, including weight scales, blood pressure/heart rate, and even pulse oximetry.

The diagnostic impressions that result from telemedicine encounters could encompass many disorders such as insomnia, circadian rhythm disorders, restless legs syndrome, and hypersomnias such as narcolepsy, in addition to sleep-disordered breathing. Educational resources could be physically mailed to patients or, more commonly, delivered electronically to supplement the visit, as typically done after an in-person visit. Cognitive behavioral therapy for insomnia (CBT-I) could be delivered via telemedicine, software applications, or web-based therapy. Actigraphs could be mailed to the patient, or the patient could pick up equipment and receive education by telephone or tele-video with the technologist. Blood tests could be ordered to evaluate for secondary causes of restless legs syndrome, with results returned to the ordering clinician. Adaptations in the continuity of care for each sleep disorder were considered, and clinical practices implemented these changes.

Sleep telemedicine proved to be an effective tool.[8] Although challenges remained in implementation, both clinicians and patients became more accustomed to this new model of care. Early survey data indicated that sleep clinicians adopted telemedicine more swiftly than their general medicine colleagues and that patients and clinicians were overall satisfied with the model.[9]

The implementation of this effective tool, however, was possible only because of major efforts by clinical practices to adapt to telemedicine. This demand for rapid adaptation affected all team members. Scheduling staff needed to provide patients with specific education around the telemedicine platform and the process. Data needed to be obtained ahead of time, including new patient questionnaires and other routine questionnaires. Rooming patients varied from one practice to another; sometimes support staff joined the telemedicine visit before the clinician to ensure that any technical issues had been resolved and that patients were prepared for their visit with an environment that included appropriate lighting and adequate safety and privacy. Other practices had no support staff, and the initial contact with the patient was performed by the clinician. Sometimes technical challenges led to delays in the start of the clinical visit. Patient check-out also needed to be modified and relied heavily on electronic messaging between clinicians and support staff as well as between clinics and patients. Some institutions implemented parallel software that integrated scheduling software, the electronic medical record, and the team's private messaging platform. Naturally, some clinicians and patients were less comfortable with this approach, and education was required. Patients who lacked access to broadband or technology were further disadvantaged and distanced from receiving medical care that was available to others; socioeconomic factors, advanced age, and physical or mental disability continued to be important social determinants of care.

The field of sleep medicine relies heavily on testing for obstructive sleep apnea (OSA). Although the trend has shifted more testing into the home since HSATs were approved in 2007, the pandemic accelerated this transition. Sleep laboratories and practices needed to adapt. In-laboratory polysomnography was generally reserved for the more severe and clinically symptomatic patients, especially those with comorbidities. HSATs were deployed to patients who could be tested at home. Sleep laboratories examined their physical spaces and incorporated physical distancing and heightened disinfection techniques. Clinical staff used personal protective equipment (PPE) routinely for in-laboratory patients and needed to reimagine the deployment of HSAT equipment. To minimize patient contact for staff, mail-order programs were developed using disposable HSAT equipment.

Adaptations to Support Fellowship Training via Telemedicine

Sleep medicine clinical fellowship training programs are usually 1 year long.[10] During the pandemic, sleep fellows needed to complete the required work to demonstrate required competencies, even as some were redirected to assist with the care of large surges in the numbers of COVID-19 patients who were seeking care in inpatient and out-patient settings. Telemedicine supported graduate medical education in a bi-directional manner. Sleep fellows used telemedicine to see patients (although this was inconsistent around the country due to reimbursement being tied to the attending in a time-based billing model), so this was not an option universally. Attendings and fellows took advantage of the fact that they could each be in a separate home- or office-based location, with the patient in a third location. When it was available, fellows received hands-on practical experience in how to conduct a telemedicine visit while also learning how to navigate through the logistics of delivering care remotely and becoming comfortable using the telemedicine platform.

Telemedicine also had a role in training the fellows; many programs developed short, on-demand videos to teach core competencies, hosted extramural guest speakers, and provided access to national podcasts, printed materials, or webinars hosted by professional societies. Telemedicine and remote learning allowed for larger numbers of visiting professors to teach fellows, as the time, expense, and inconvenience of travel were eliminated. The ability to enlarge the screen, freeze frames, and focus on key examination findings could allow learners access to in-depth examination findings with their supervising physician.

Telemedicine allowed an expansion of attending supervision in novel ways while incorporating a patient-centered experience. Patients who preferred or required in-person assessment could be seen by a fellow at a practice site, with the virtual addition of supervising attending physicians to review, assess, confirm, or add to the history and examination and to contribute to management and teaching, as would occur during in-person teaching. Such flexibility, which is due to expire with the end of the pandemic declaration, may have incentivized teaching faculty to continue to engage with trainees. Some facilities also used telemedicine to supervise physician assistants and nurse practitioners, although the legal requirements for this varied among states.

The Fundamental Role of Telemedicine Reimbursement and the Relaxation of Regulations

Widespread telemedicine expansion in clinical and educational arenas, which resulted in access to care and support of educational goals in sleep medicine, was only possible because of an urgent, significant change in reimbursement and the relaxation of regulations. In March 2020,[11] the CMS opted to permit reimbursement for telemedicine services, on parity with in-person visits, even when both clinicians and patients were at home. Along with this were varying degrees of reciprocity of licensure and waiving formal licensure in some states in favor of temporary licenses. Some of the waivers included only clinicians who would work in another state taking care of COVID-19 patients. Other states had broad waivers allowing for telemedicine to take place across state borders without formal licensure. Most critical was the allowance of payment parity for telemedicine and relaxation of what constituted a telemedicine visit, namely, that although audio and video were preferred, some patients could be evaluated using audio alone, and these visits would still be reimbursed. Available estimates suggest that payment facilitated access and continuation of care during the pandemic for millions of patients with sleep disorders.

Specific to sleep medicine clinics, there was also a lifting of the requirements to have a face-to-face visit before prescribing PAP therapy. This lightened the clinical burden for sleep clinicians, many of whom were being deployed to work in COVID-19 units. Reimbursement for remote patient monitoring remains in its infancy in our field.

What Have We Learned?

According to an AASM pulse survey,[6] sleep clinicians transitioned to telemedicine quickly and in higher percentages than other subspecialties. Sleep medicine was well-suited to telemedicine evaluations. Yurcheshen et al.[12] compared in-person clinic visits to remote visits and found that information gathering and the ability to order the appropriate test were not different between the two. Further analysis from multiple sources confirmed high patient and clinician satisfaction for telemedicine clinic visits.[9] Many experts have indicated that telemedicine will endure, including a former administrator of CMS[13] during the COVID-19 pandemic. Investments in infrastructure and ongoing viable reimbursement models are needed for telemedicine to continue and for patient and clinician experiences to improve. Ongoing training must occur at multiple levels, including sleep medicine fellows. Their training in telemedicine has been hampered in some regions due to an inability to bill for time spent by the fellow in addition to the attending physician. Some rural areas have been limited by poor access to broadband, thus further disenfranchising rural patients who are already in so-called "health deserts." Further consideration should focus on identifying gaps in care, both from a socioeconomic standpoint and through a technology literacy lens.

Where Do We Go From Here?

The pandemic caused rapid shifts in routine. Many of the solutions were rushed and reactive. It is imperative to consider these changes as initial ones, rather than temporary ones. Further improvement must occur on many levels, including infrastructure; patient technology literacy, access to technology, and robust broadband; improved health literacy; and assessment of long-term outcomes of these changes on patients, the health care workforce, and medical education.

COVID-19 has created new medical disorders and worsened existing ones. Long-term effects of COVID-19 on sleep in particular must be investigated. This involves creation of a long COVID-19 registry and collecting data for epidemiological purposes and future research. Many health care facilities have created long COVID-19 clinics,[14] often multidisciplinary, to address the myriad of symptoms that accompany long COVID-19. Some sleep disorders, including those of central nervous system hypersomnolence, may be associated with long COVID-19.[15]

Telemedicine staff will need to be educated about best practices. This involves an analysis of conditions suitable for a telemedicine visit rather than an in-person visit. Enhanced patient examination tools may be accessible in the future, such as digital otoscopes[16] or stethoscopes that are currently marketed toward health care consumers and use smartphones to display images or sound data that are collected. Patients have proven to be adept in appropriate positioning and lighting to enhance the physical examination once they have received the appropriate training. As telemedicine processes continue to mature, patients are likely to have more familiarity with all of these components.

Sleep medicine has long suffered from an underappreciation of its role in promoting mental and physical health due to cultural factors. Many people undervalue sleep and may avoid seeking sleep health care. In fact, such cultural attitudes may at least partly explain why 80% of OSA cases remain undiagnosed.[17] Because patients are typically encouraged to seek sleep services by their bed partners, many are ambivalent and may decide not to pursue evaluation due to the need for time and travel. Telemedicine has not only reduced the need for travel, but it has also allowed access to specialist care, thus improving access for both the patient and caregiver. In addition to reducing the need for time and travel, remote patient visits have removed many other traditional barriers that compound the reluctance to seek help; these include physical or mental disabilities or socioeconomic limitations that make travel difficult, such as lack of access to affordable transportation or parking. Other expenses, such as family care and time away from work, can also be reduced when telemedicine is used in place of in-person care.

Consumer sleep technology (CST) may allow for the capture of longitudinal data. These technologies can provide pulse oximetry or heart rate variability, can estimate sleep and wakefulness, and have already proven to be helpful in measuring "off-PAP" sleep time.[18] CST provides OSA awareness, which may prompt health care consumers to seek clinical evaluation. CST is ubiquitous, and patients are typically comfortable with such technology. Telemedicine is an ideal way for patients who have identified a potential sleep concern via their CST to then have a face-to-face synchronous evaluation by a sleep specialist.

Supporting telemedicine legislation and advocacy will help ensure longevity of this essential tool. This advocacy can be on an individual basis by directly contacting legislators or by becoming active in professional societies that advocate for telemedicine reimbursement to ensure that this valuable tool remains viable. We must continue to improve telemedicine platforms, ensuring that they remain patient-friendly and secure, while also reducing time and cognitive demand on health care providers. Reimbursement must continue and must include payment parity compared with in-person visits. Many clinics invested heavily in new equipment and platforms and must receive appropriate reimbursement.

The recent COVID-19 pandemic was a disruptor within health care unlike any others. Although the pandemic highlighted existing disparities in health care access, it also allowed telemedicine to reduce some of these barriers to care. Future growth of telemedicine must examine how to improve care delivery to marginalized individuals and to those without ready access to technology. Perhaps a hybrid approach combining some in-person visits with remote visits could be considered. Another consideration would be to improve access to technology by providing it via a private booth in a public library or other publicly accessible, yet private location. Above all, the lessons learned from this recent pandemic must not be forgotten. We must continue to improve access to care and take heed not to further disenfranchise those already marginalized. As sleep is foundational for good health, an investment in ways to continue to improve access to sleep health care would have wide-ranging, beneficial impact on the health and safety of all individuals.

References

1. Choo EK, Strehlow M, Del Rios M, et al. Observational study of organisational responses of 17 US hospitals over the first year of the COVID-19 pandemic. *BMJ Open*. 2023;13(5):e067986.
2. Hamner L, Dubbel P, Capron I, et al. High SARS-CoV-2 attack rate following exposure at a choir practice—Skagit County, Washington, March 2020. https://www.cdc.gov/mmwr/volumes/69/wr/mm6919e6.htm. Accessed March 1, 2024.
3. Lu J, Gu J, Li K, et al. COVID-19 outbreak associated with air conditioning in restaurant, Guangzhou, China, 2020. https://wwwnc.cdc.gov/eid/article/26/7/20-0764_article. Accessed March 1, 2024.
4. Roxby AC, Greninger AL, Hatfield KM, et al. Outbreak Investigation of COVID-19 Among Residents and Staff of an Independent and Assisted Living Community for Older Adults in Seattle, Washington. *JAMA Intern Med*. 2020;180(8):1101–1105. doi:10.1001/jamainternmed.2020.2233
5. McMichael TM, Clark S, Pogosjans S, et al. COVID-19 in a long-term care facility—King County, Washington, February 27–March 9, 2020. https://www.cdc.gov/mmwr/volumes/69/wr/mm6912e1.htm. Accessed March 1, 2024.
6. Ramar K. AASM takes the pulse of the sleep field and responds to COVID-19. J Clin Sleep Med. 2020;16(11):1939–1942. https://doi.org/10.5664/jcsm.8846. https://aasm.org/covid-19-resources/coronavirus-pulse-survey-sleep/. Accessed March 1, 2024.
7. Johnson KG, Sullivan SS, Nti A, et al. The impact of the COVID-19 pandemic on sleep medicine practices. *J Clin Sleep Med*. 2021;17(1):79-87. https://aasm.org/covid-19-resources/coronavirus-pulse-survey-sleep/. Accessed March 1, 2024.
8. Shamim-Uzzaman QA, Bae CJ, Ehsan Z, et al. The use of telemedicine for the diagnosis and treatment of sleep disorders: an American Academy of Sleep Medicine update. *J Clin Sleep Med*. 2021;17(5):1103-1107.
9. Ramaswamy A, Yu M, Drangsholt S, et al. Patient satisfaction with telemedicine during the COVID-19 pandemic: retrospective cohort study. *J Med Internet Res*. 2020;22(9):e20786.
10. ABIM. Sleep Medicine Policies. https://www.abim.org/certification/policies/internal-medicine-subspecialty-policies/sleep-medicine.aspx. [Accessed 19 December 2023].
11. CMS Telehealth. https://www.cms.gov/Medicare/Medicare-General-Information/Telehealth. [Accessed 12 December 2023].
12. Yurcheshen ME, Pigeon W, Marcus CZ, et al. Interrater reliability between in-person and telemedicine evaluations in obstructive sleep apnea. *J Clin Sleep Med*. 2021;17(7):1435-1440.
13. Dyrda L. 'The genie's out of the bottle on this one': Seema Verma hints at the future of telehealth for CMS beneficiaries. https://www.beckershospitalreview.com/telehealth/the-genie-s-out-of-the-bottle-on-this-one-seema-verma-hints-at-the-future-of-telehealth-for-cms-beneficiaries.html. Accessed March 1, 2024.
14. Respiratory Health Association. Long COVID Clinics by State. https://resphealth.org/wp-content/uploads/2022/12/Long-COVID-Clinics-Final-1.pdf. Accessed March 1, 2024.
15. Sarkanen T, Partinen M, Bjorvatn B, et al. Association between hypersomnolence and the COVID-19 pandemic: The International COVID-19 Sleep Study (ICOSS). *Sleep Medicine*. 2023;107:108–115. doi:10.1016/j.sleep.2023.04.024. https://aasm.org/covid-19-resources/coronavirus-pulse-survey-sleep/. Accessed March 1, 2024.
16. Amazon Digital Otoscopes. https://www.amazon.com/Otoscope-Anykit-Rechargeable-Supports-Recording/dp/B081DF1DGZ/ref=asc_df_B081DF1DGZ/?tag=hyprod-20&linkCode=df0&hvadid=50779014665 1&hvpos=&hvnetw=g&hvrand=4245377498176245856&hvpone=&hvptwo=&hvqmt=&hvdev=c&hvd vcmdl=&hvlocint=&hvlocphy=9020213&hvtargid=pla-905324313295&psc=1. [Accessed 19 December 2023.].
17. American Academy of Sleep Medicine. Economic Impact of Obstructive Sleep Apnea. https://aasm.org/advocacy/initiatives/economic-impact-obstructive-sleep-apnea/. Accessed 19 December 2023.
18. Thomas RJ, Bianchi MT Urgent need to improve PAP management: the devil is in two (fixable) details. *J Clin Sleep Med*. 2017;13(5):657–664. https://www.beckershospitalreview.com/telehealth/the-genie-s-out-of-the-bottle-on-this-one-seema-verma-hints-at-the-future-of-telehealth-for-cms-beneficiaries.html. Accessed March 1, 2024.

Implementation of Telemedicine

CHAPTER 3

Regulatory and Ethical Considerations in Sleep Telemedicine

Janet Hilbert ■ Barry Fields

A History of Telemedicine Regulation and Terminology

Modern telemedicine commenced in the early 1990s when the Internet and other technology were integrated to promote long-distance health care. But as this new modality developed, so too did attempts to regulate it. Regulations arose as never-before-seen procedural and ethical quandaries developed, such as how to license physicians and other health care providers who care for patients outside of their states and how to reimburse those practitioners for their patient encounters. Only five states had enacted any rules related to telemedicine in 1992.[1] Early recognition of this deficiency came in a 1995 analysis of state telemedicine policies. Data from that year revealed that "Only 3 states have addressed the provider licensure issue…Few states have addressed another issue critical to the future of telemedicine—reimbursement. The only significant policymaking has been in Louisiana."[2] Telemedicine regulation outside of the United States was equally underdeveloped, even precarious. One British author in 1995 noted, "unforeseen medico-legal implications of telemedicine will be revealed by litigation as it arises."[3]

TERMINOLOGY: TELEHEALTH VS. TELEMEDICINE

An enduring hurdle to telemedicine regulation has been imprecise terminology, even regarding the term *telemedicine* itself. An early and quickly propagated definition of telemedicine arose from an Institute of Medicine statement in 1996. They defined it as "the use of electronic information and communications technologies to provide and support health care when distance separates the participant."[4] This definition is notable for its breadth in at least two regards. First, no specific form of communication was excluded; telephone-only interaction fell within this definition. Second, it does not limit telemedicine to provider-patient interactions. That is, health care–focused meetings or conferences could fall within this definition. Furthermore, often interchangeable terminology such as *telehealth* was not defined.

Despite its importance, this distinction between *telemedicine* and *telehealth* has proven elusive. Clarity has emerged (somewhat) over the past quarter century. As noted in Figure 3.1, telehealth is now applied more generally to the broader aspects of that early telemedicine definition, with the Health Resources and Services Administration (HRSA) defining it as "the use of electronic information and telecommunications technologies to support long-distance clinical health care, patient and professional health-related education, public health and health administration."[5] Telemedicine usually implies direct clinical care, but with remote patient and health care practitioner interaction. The Federation of State Medical Boards defines it as "the practice of medicine

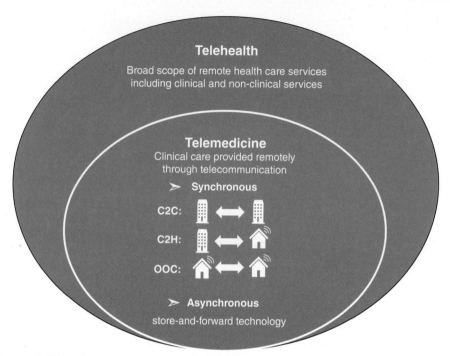

Figure 3.1   What is telemedicine? *C2C,* Center-to-center; *C2H,* center-to-home; *OOC,* out-of-center.

using electronic communications, information technology, or other means between a licensee in one location, and a patient in another location, with or without an intervening health care provider."[6] The American Academy of Sleep Medicine's (AASM's) Sleep Telemedicine Implementation Guide supports this distinction for sleep medicine.[7] Therefore we use the *telemedicine* terminology for this chapter.

REGULATION EVOLUTION

Like the very definition of telemedicine, American state-based telemedicine regulations evolved steadily through first two decades of the 21st century. More and more states developed medical care payer "parity laws." Telemedicine visits could be reimbursed at equivalent levels to in-person visits, albeit with somewhat variable, state-specific definitions as to what constitutes "telemedicine."[8] Similarly, an Interstate Medical Licensure Compact (IMLC) has grown to facilitate cross-border licensing in more states since 2017 (discussed later).[9] From its inception, it has been up to states to decide whether to join the IMLC. However, where states' regulations progressed and modernized, U.S. federal regulations remained relatively stagnant. The Centers for Medicare and Medicaid Services (CMS) continued its policy of tight geographic and demographic restrictions on who could receive telemedicine-based care and how they could receive it.[10] Furthermore, significant restrictions in Internet-based prescribing negatively affected sleep telemedicine feasibility. The Ryan Haight Online Pharmacy Consumer Protection Act of 2008 specified that a physician must have at least one in-person visit with a patient before issuing that individual a valid prescription. Although the Act contained a provision that excused telemedicine physicians from this rule, a registration process to operationalize this exception was never created.[11]

THE COVID-19 PANDEMIC

Early in 2019, the American College of Physicians stated, "As payers, both private and public, begin establishing guidelines and paying for telehealth services, most expect this area to explode in the next year or two."[12] Their statement was more prophetic than anyone could have known. As the coronavirus disease 2019 (COVID-19) pandemic spread the next year, some aspects of telemedicine regulation loosened in the United States and around the world. For instance, in March 2020, the CMS announced that telemedicine visits would be reimbursable even if patients did not live in federally defined health care shortage areas.[13] Additionally, many states have loosened interstate licensing requirements to improve medical care access within their state.[10]

Although these changes are officially temporary, their impact on sleep telemedicine will likely be long-lasting. Beyond policies altering regulations on reimbursement and licensing, the COVID-19 pandemic has changed telemedicine-related terminology itself. Until 2020, the main form of telemedicine was center-to-center (C2C), where health care practitioners (distant site) and patients (originating site) are in clinical locations (see Figure 3.1). Some telemedicine was conducted in a center-to-home (C2H) format, where an originating site could be a patient's home while receiving care from a practitioner at a distant clinical site. Notably, most of these visits were not Medicare reimbursable before 2020. Since the commencement of the COVID-19 pandemic, out-of-center (OOC) telemedicine has become more widespread. In this modality, neither the originating site nor the distant site needs to be clinical. OOC telemedicine's future feasibility will depend on the fate of temporary, COVID-19–related regulatory alterations.

Telemedicine Regulation Resources

One of the few constants in telemedicine regulation over the past several decades has been change, and never has this truth been so apparent as during the COVID-19 pandemic. Indeed, any description of local, state, and federal policies is solely a point-in-time assertion with questionable validity in the not-too-distant future. Therefore, though the broad brush strokes of telemedicine regulation will be described later in this chapter, discussing resources for the most up-to-date information rather than listing particular details appears prudent.

Table 3.1 lists major resources for information about sleep and general telemedicine. The list is not exhaustive, but it provides useful references for up-to-date information. Organizations are accompanied by their telemedicine-focused websites, which are updated regularly as "living documents" of the time. If the reader is an AASM member, a helpful first step is reviewing resources through the AASM telemedicine page[14]; several of the other resources in Table 3.1 are accessible from that web page. These resources not only provide answers to questions but also provide *what questions to ask* in an organized format. For instance, one might not realize malpractice insurance rules vary when it comes to telemedicine, how to find that information, and so on.

Once questions pertinent to sleep telemedicine regulations are generated, several resources in Table 3.1 provide up-to-date overviews of current telemedicine regulatory status. The Center for Connected Health Policy (CCHP) is a particularly helpful source for details about state-by-state topics such as payer laws, licensing guidelines, and rules regarding consent for telemedicine care provision.[15] The American Telemedicine Association (ATA) provides similar content, as well as a "tracker" of ongoing national and state telehealth legislation.[16] The HRSA is another comprehensive resource focused on policy at the national level.[17]

More focused resources include the CMS telehealth website, which details federal reimbursement policy and displays the annual physician fee schedule.[15] The IMLC website provides current information about interstate licensing,[9] while the Rural Information Hub targets rural programs.[18] Although this chapter is focused on U.S. telemedicine regulations, Table 3.1 also provides resources for other

TABLE 3.1 ■ Useful Resources

United States	International
American Academy of Sleep Medicine: https://www.aasm.org/clinical-resources/ telemedicine/ American Telemedicine Association: https://www.americantelemed.org/ American Medical Association: https://www.ama-assn.org/ Centers for Medicare and Medicaid Services: https://www.cms.gov/Medicare/Medicare- General-Information/Telehealth Center for Connected Health Policy: https://www.cchpca.org/ Interstate Medical Licensure Compact: https://www.imlcc.org Health Resources and Services Administration: https://telehealth.hhs.gov/ Rural Health Information Hub: https://www.ruralhealthinfo.org/toolkits/telehealth/	Australian Department of Health https://www.health.gov.au/news/health-alerts/ novel-coronavirus-2019-ncov-health-alert/ coronavirus-covid-19-advice-for-the-health-and- disability-sector/providing-health-care-remotely- during-covid-19 Canadian Medical Association: https://www.cma.ca/ The Canadian Medical Protective Association: https://www.cmpa-acpm.ca/en/membership/ protection-for-members/principles-of-assistance/ practising-telehealth National Health Service (England, UK): https://www.england.nhs.uk/tecs/

parts of the world. Like the American resources, they provide up-to-date information in the rapidly changing telemedicine landscape. The United Kingdom's National Health Service website is particularly illustrative of how telemedicine is regulated within a national health system.[19]

Telemedicine Regulation Domains and Descriptions

Telemedicine regulation can seem a complex tangle of federal, state, and local policies all existing and interacting in a rapidly changing environment. This chapter is not meant to perpetuate that complexity; on the contrary, we seek to organize regulations into four broad domains, describe relevant concepts, and provide context for the more detailed information available from resources in Table 3.1.

Figure 3.2 shows those four domains of telemedicine regulation, with components of each domain noted and described further. Individuals or organizations developing or sustaining a sleep telemedicine program must continually revisit licensing, privacy and security, clinical care, and medico-legal regulations as they pertain to their practice. This iterative process, signified with the circular arrows at the center of Figure 3.2, should be conducted in accordance with up-to-date material present in Table 3.1 resources and any other policies provided to them locally.

LICENSING

State Licensure

Licensing requirements vary considerably by state, but practitioners (distant site) generally must be licensed in the state in which patients are located at the time of the visit (originating site).[11] Telemedicine encounters are subject to regulatory and documentation requirements, similar to in-person encounters. Scope of practice may or may not be the same in telemedicine and in-person encounters. For example, some states may restrict the ordering of tests or durable medical equipment (DME) without a physical examination.[20]

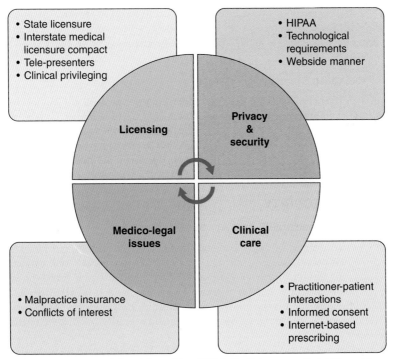

Figure 3.2 Regulatory aspects of sleep telemedicine. *HIPAA,* Health Insurance Portability and Accountability Act of 1996.

Telemedicine policy changes have occurred frequently during the COVID-19 public health emergency. The CMS broadened access to telehealth services.[13] Most states incorporated waivers to allow for the care of patients during the public health emergency, but there is considerable variability in services and practitioners that are covered by these waivers. These waivers often have not been incorporated into permanent policy.[21] The CCHP is an excellent resource for updates on state and federal policy changes.[15]

Interstate Medical Licensure Compact

The IMLC is an agreement among states to streamline the licensing process for physicians who wish to practice in multiple states. It is a voluntary, expedited pathway to licensure for physicians who qualify.[9] As of this writing, the Compact includes 29 states, the District of Columbia, and Guam. Physicians who qualify can complete one application and obtain separate licenses from participating states. States can expedite licensing by sharing information submitted in the state of principal licensure. Participating states and physician qualifications are listed on the IMLC website.

Similar to the IMLC, a Nurse Licensure Compact (NLC) allows nurses to practice in other NLC states.[22] State regulations also determine the scope of practice for polysomnographic technologists and respiratory therapists.[20] Interstate polysomnographic technologist licensing requirements are variable, and state policy should be consulted.[11]

Tele-presenters

In the C2C model of telemedicine, tele-presenters at the originating site aid in navigating patients through the technical aspects of the visit and may assist with physical examination. States vary in whether tele-presenters are necessary for the visit to occur, what type of medical provider may fill the role of tele-presenter, and whether the tele-presenter must be in the room with the patient during the encounter or simply available on the premises.[7] State policy should be consulted for guidance.

Clinical Privileging

All practitioners (including telemedicine practitioners) must be credentialed and maintain clinical privileges at the health care facilities in which they practice. The burden on both the health care institutions and practitioners is thus potentially increased in telemedicine. Some hospitals or health care facilities may choose to utilize a credentialing by proxy process that is approved by the CMS. To do so, the originating health care institution, the distant health care institution, and the practitioner must meet specific criteria.[23]

PRIVACY AND SECURITY

Health Insurance Portability and Accountability Act

The Health Insurance Portability and Accountability Act of 1996 (HIPAA) provides data privacy and security provisions to safeguard medical information.[24] The privacy rule protects patient medical records and identifiable health information, while the security rule covers confidentiality, integrity, and availability of electronic protected health information (ePHI). The approach to protected health information is the same during telemedicine visits as it is for in-person visits. HIPAA requirements as well as state privacy, confidentiality, security, and medical retention rules should be met.[20]

HIPAA guidelines on telemedicine stipulate that (1) only authorized users should have access to ePHI, (2) a system of secure communication should be implemented to protect the integrity of ePHI, and (3) a system of monitoring communications containing ePHI should be implemented to prevent accidental or malicious breaches. Additionally, a medical practitioner or a health care organization creating ePHI that is stored by a third party is required to have a business associate agreement with the party storing the data.[25]

Given the rapid deployment of telemedicine during the COVID-19 public health emergency, the U.S. Department of Health and Human Services stipulated that "Covered health care providers will not be subject to penalties for violations of the HIPAA Privacy, Security, and Breach Notification Rules that occur in the good faith provision of telehealth during the COVID-19 nationwide public health emergency."[26]

Technological Requirements

Technological features can help ensure HIPAA compliance.[8] Communication and data storage systems should be encrypted, and devices/platforms should be password- or biometric-protected.[27] Hardware and software should be up to date with regular security updates. Applications used to provide telemedicine services may require HIPAA business associate agreements. Audio and video recording are discouraged due to hacking concerns. Access to telemedicine systems should be restricted to authorized users only (with unauthorized access attempts reviewable). Data stored in other platforms (e.g., sleep testing software, positive airway pressure data platforms) and incorporated into the electronic medical record must be secure.[11] See Chapter 18 for more specific recommendations.

Webside Manner

See Chapter 9 for further information. Practitioner actions before, during, and after the patient encounter can also help ensure HIPPA compliance (see Chapter 9). In addition to conducting telemedicine encounters in private settings, best practices include use of headphones and/or computer privacy screens if needed to ensure patient privacy, inactivity timeout functions, and password protection.

CLINICAL CARE

Practitioner-Patient Interactions (See Chapter 8)

Defining how practitioners interact with patients through telemedicine is important to understanding clinical care–focused regulation. Many states and the federal government define the style of these interactions that constitutes telemedicine; this is usually in the context of permitted services for reimbursement. For instance, Georgia Medicaid defines *telemedicine* as "the use of two-way, real time interactive communication equipment to exchange the patient information from one site to another via an electronic communication system. This includes audio and video communications equipment."[28] Connecticut Medicaid's definition is very similar: "Telemedicine means the use of interactive audio, interactive video or interactive data communication in the delivery of medical advice, diagnosis, care or treatment...Telemedicine does not include the use of facsimile or audio-only telephone."[28] Regulations do not prevent practitioners from making medical decisions over the telephone or prescribe medication based on those decisions (especially if that individual has seen that patient in person before). Instead, it is the option to *charge* for that encounter that receives the most regulatory attention.

There is growing evidence that telemedicine-based sleep apnea care is not inferior to in-person care in terms of clinical outcomes, treatment adherence, or patient satisfaction.[29] That said, telemedicine as a health care delivery tool is not optimal for all patients. As discussed in the "Ethical Considerations" section later in this chapter, patients should be given complete information about what a telemedicine visit entails. This disclosure allows them to exercise autonomy in the telemedicine versus in-person medicine decision-making process. Practitioners may also deem patients to be poor candidates for initial evaluation through telemedicine based on initial complaint (e.g., a neurologically focused sleep disturbance) or audiovisual disability. Therefore choosing which patients should be treated through telemedicine is based more on personal and institutional considerations than any particular regulation; systematic exclusion of patients from telemedicine services must be avoided.

Internet-Based Prescribing

Please see Chapter 10 for more information. Regulations concerning Internet-based medication prescribing arose from cases of patient harm due to medications or treatments prescribed over the Internet by practitioners who had never physically evaluated the patient.[30] Although states' and institutions' Internet-based prescribing strategies vary,[28] there are federal regulations governing this area. The Ryan Haight Online Pharmacy Consumer Protection Act of 2008 states that prescriptions are only "valid" if the prescriber has performed at least one in-person medication evaluation of the patient.[31] Anticipating the detrimental impact this rule might have on telemedicine, the Act also states, "The Attorney General may issue to a practitioner a special registration to engage in the practice of telemedicine," thus implying an exception for patients receiving their care wholly through telemedicine. However, this special registration clause was not operationalized.

Since the COVID-19 pandemic commenced, federal regulation of Internet-based prescribing has loosened considerably. Starting in March 2020 and for the duration of the public health emergency, Internet-based prescribing (including controlled substances) is allowed as long as clinical care occurs through real-time audiovisual telemedicine.[32] It should be noted that these loosened restrictions last only as long as the public health emergency; there is still no *permanent* provision for special telemedicine practitioners to prescribe over the Internet without having first examined the patient in person.

Informed Consent

There are no federal regulations stipulating that informed consent be obtained for telemedicine encounters for them to be reimbursed through Medicare. However, many states do invoke this requirement before their Medicaid funds may be accessed. The frequency with which informed consent should be obtained (e.g., before only the initial clinical encounter or before every encounter) differs among states. Updated state policies should be consulted.[15] Similarly, private insurers may have informed consent stipulations. Because not all payors have these informed consent requirements, it is up to practitioners to familiarize themselves with these rules.

Beyond documenting informed consent for the sake of reimbursement, practitioners may find it part of their institutional culture (or even a requirement) to obtain consent before beginning a telemedicine encounter. There is no accepted format for a telemedicine encounter consent form; the Agency for Healthcare Research and Quality provides one straightforward example.[33] Nevertheless, informed consent need not imply that the patient releases the practitioner from any harm that may result from the encounter. That is, informed consent for telemedicine is not a *medical release* as may be utilized for a surgical procedure.

MEDICO-LEGAL ISSUES

Malpractice Insurance

As of the writing of this chapter, there has never been successful litigation of a practitioner simply because telemedicine was utilized. Nevertheless, the same liabilities may arise during telemedicine encounters as during in-person encounters if standards of care are not upheld. There are no federal or state policies regulating whether or how malpractice insurers should cover telemedicine. Therefore it is up to the practitioner to ensure that any malpractice insurance covers (1) care at the originating and distant sites and (2) the telemedicine modality practiced (C2C, C2H, OOC). In some cases, supplemental coverage may be needed.[34]

Like many areas of telemedicine, the COVID-19 pandemic has led to renewed focus on this malpractice insurance application. Current guidance suggests contacting one's malpractice insurer to ensure the appropriate coverage described earlier is in effect.[35] Insurers typically require compliance with all applicable local, state, and federal regulations. If an insurance claim is filed, plaintiff attorneys will likely ascertain if all regulations were followed, such as intrastate medical licensure or licensure waivers. It is best not to assume that an originating site's state has relaxed intrapandemic regulations to the same extent as a distant site. Health care professionals must still do their due diligence to ensure that they are not exposing themselves to unforeseen liability.

CONFLICTS OF INTEREST

Conflicts of interest—real or perceived—can occur within telemedicine as they do with in-person care. These conflicts usually arise when a practitioner is positioned to receive financial gain when a patient utilizes a good or service. A review by Venkateshiah et al. effectively splits federal conflict of interest regulations into two categories: (1) self-referral prohibition and (2) anti-kickback.[20] The self-referral prohibition rules, also called the Stark Laws, prohibit practitioners from receiving Medicare reimbursement for goods and services with which the practitioner has a financial relationship. A common example within sleep medicine is DME provision; Medicare will not reimburse a practitioner for sleep apnea equipment if that individual owns or has a financial link to the DME provider. Similar restrictions typically apply to telemedicine equipment and services, thus discouraging practitioners from self-referral if they have a financial interest in an equipment manufacturer, service provider, and so on. However, the COVID-19 pandemic–associated public health emergency has generated exceptions to these laws.[36] Practitioners in this situation (i.e., potentially profiting from both telemedicine clinical care *and* a telemedicine business) should consult CMS and perhaps an attorney for updated regulations.[37] Since the Stark Law is a federal regulation, it only applies to federal reimbursement.

Anti-kickback regulations generally cover more egregious criminal activity, while the Stark Laws are *civil* laws, and the federal Anti-Kickback Statute is a *criminal* statute. It "prohibits offering, paying, soliciting, or receiving anything of value to induce or reward referrals or generate federal health care program business."[20] As it relates to this chapter, practitioners are prohibited from purchasing telemedicine equipment for an outside provider or hospital with the implication that the entity will then refer to that practitioner exclusively for all sleep-related services.[11] Federal Anti-Kickback Statute violations are punishable by steep fines and/or imprisonment. State anti-kickback statutes may also apply, bringing their own set of professional and legal repercussions. Although neither these statutes nor the Stark Laws apply specifically to telemedicine, they will undoubtedly be invoked more in this realm as the field continues to grow.

Ethical Considerations

Although federal and local regulations are designed to help promote health care quality while controlling cost, it is ultimately up to the practitioner to ensure that patients receive appropriate care for their specific situation. It is within this milieu—balancing telemedicine advantages and limitations with patient needs—that ethical dilemmas exist; they have only grown more widespread with sleep telemedicine's recent proliferation. Ethics pillars pertaining to telemedicine are the same as those domains applied to any other area of medicine. Namely, practitioners must be sure to maintain patient autonomy, beneficence, nonmaleficence, and justice. A summary of these principles appears in Figure 3.3.

AUTONOMY

Autonomy refers to patients' rights to make their own decisions about their medical care. As this principle applies telemedicine, patients must be informed enough about the telemedicine visit to choose (1) whether they wish to proceed with telemedicine versus in-person care and (2) the style of telemedicine in which they wish to participate (i.e., clinical video telehealth or telephone). Although technology limitations and disease complexity can present inherent restrictions on these visit venues, patient autonomy can be supported through education to help them make decisions that *are* within their control. Scheduling staff may describe what a telemedicine

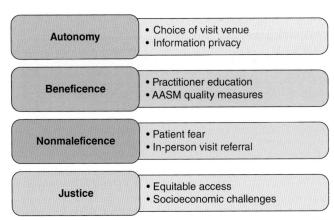

Figure 3.3 Ethical considerations in sleep telemedicine. *AASM,* American Academy of Sleep Medicine.

experience entails, or other sleep team members could explain the benefits and risks of telemedicine given the patient's clinical situation. Clinical staff are also responsible for maintaining patients' information privacy, another key element in supporting their autonomy. Medical information should be treated with the same security as during any other visit, and any individuals present with the patient (originating site) or with the practitioner (distant site) should be identified. Patient's comfort with these other individuals' presence should be ascertained at the start of the clinical encounter.[38] Any unauthorized access to patients' health information at either site of the interaction can erode their autonomy in making medical decisions.

BENEFICENCE

Beneficence describes a practitioner's duty to benefit patients in all situations, and they can fulfill that duty partly through education. The rising tide of telemedicine has brought with it many new technical, regulatory, and ethical considerations not previously encountered. Sleep medicine has lagged behind other specialties (dermatology, emergency medicine, neurology) in formalizing telemedicine education.[11] If sleep practitioners are to provide the most beneficial care, it behooves them to review material such as this textbook and the references in Table 3.1 for the most up-to-date telemedicine techniques and guidelines. When these practitioners wish to compare their quality of care with national standards, they might also reference a series of Quality Measures, published by the AASM and easily adaptable to telemedicine. For instance, the Quality Measures for the Care of Adult Patients with Obstructive Sleep Apnea (OSA) suggest assessment of OSA treatment adherence as an important Process Measure.[39] Sleep telemedicine clinics can easily adapt this Measure to their style of care; most PAP machines come with wireless download capability, and treatment adherence is easily viewable for both patients and practitioners via the Internet. Telemedicine software's "screen-sharing" capabilities can allow both individuals to view the data simultaneously as part of a C2C, C2H, or OOC telemedicine encounter. These adaptations allow telemedicine clinics the same Process Measure attainment capabilities as in-person clinics. In doing so, they help ensure that patient beneficence remains firmly intact.

NONMALEFICENCE

Nonmaleficence refers to a practitioner's duty not to harm the patient and/or society over the course of medical care. Although the idea of telemedicine may first appeal to patients, the reality of new technology, logistics, and contact with a new provider far away may instill a sense of concern—even fear—in patients. These issues can be ameliorated through patient education and reassurance that in-person visits are still possible (though in-person visits themselves come with other potentially stressful factors such as travel and limited access). Additionally, sleep practitioners must recognize when in-person care is more appropriate for further follow-up, whether due to patient disability (hearing or visual impairment) or need for more detailed evaluation (e.g., neurological or oral examination). Referral to an in-person provider closer to the patient may effectively terminate the patient's relationship with the telemedicine provider. However, this action supports the ethical principle of nonmaleficence when undertaken for the direct benefit of the patient.[40]

JUSTICE

Justice is upheld when a practitioner ensures fairness in medical access and decisions among all patients. Although every patient should have access to sleep telemedicine, practitioner supply vastly outstrips patient demand. The AASM estimates that there are approximately 43,000 Americans for every 1 board-certified sleep specialist. Furthermore, most of these specialists are clustered in relatively few states such as New York, Florida, Texas, and California.[41] Although telemedicine can make more equitable distribution possible, regulatory considerations (described earlier) and time limitations prove formidable hurdles. That is, just because practitioners *can* conduct visits through telemedicine does not guarantee that they have the schedule availability to do so. Socioeconomic factors can also erode patients' equitable access to telemedicine. Although about 80% of Americans have access to a smart phone and 75% of them have broadband Internet access, those percentages are reduced for individuals with lower income and educational attainment levels.[42] Because these individuals are also most likely to experience disparate health care compared with more affluent socioeconomic groups, telemedicine does not necessarily promote justice in receiving this care. It behooves any sleep telemedicine practitioner to remain aware of these disparities when designing and sustaining more inclusive clinical programs.

Conclusion

Sleep telemedicine is a useful *tool* to enhance access to sleep medicine care. But like any tool, it should be utilized in the appropriate setting by individuals who know how to use it within the current regulatory landscape. Telemedicine has been feasible for decades, but various regulations contributed to its sluggish deployment; it took the COVID-19 pandemic to showcase its great utility and true promise. How temporarily relaxed regulations will predict permanent policy reform is yet to be determined, but as former CMS administrator Seema Verma said, "There's absolutely no going back."[43] Therefore looking forward and not back, it is important to stay abreast of rapidly evolving changes in telemedicine regulations (see Table 3.1). Yet even as telemedicine regulation evolves, the medical ethics underpinning it stay the same. These principles will continue to endure no matter what the future holds for sleep telemedicine. It is up to sleep practitioners to uphold these standards as telemedicine takes an ever-firmer foothold in the field.

References

1. Waller M, Stotler C. Telemedicine: a primer. *Curr Allergy Asthma Rep*. 2018;18(10):54.
2. Lipson LR, Henderson TM. State initiatives to promote telemedicine. *Telemed J*. 1996;2(2):109-121.
3. Brahams D. The medicolegal implications of teleconsulting in the UK. *J Telemed Telecare*. 1995;1(4): 196-201.
4. Institute of Medicine (US) Committee on Evaluating Clinical Applications of Telemedicine, Field MJ, ed. *Telemedicine: A Guide to Assessing Telecommunications in Health Care*. Washington DC: National Academies Press; 1996.
5. Health Resources and Services Administration. Telehealth Programs. Updated January 2021. Available at: https://www.hrsa.gov/rural-health/telehealth. Accessed March 1, 2024.
6. Federation of State Medical Boards. House of Delegates Annual Business Meeting. Updated April 28, 2018. Available at: https://www.fsmb.org/siteassets/annual-meeting/hod/april-28-2018-fsmb-hod-book. pdf. Accessed March 1, 2024.
7. American Academy of Sleep Medicine. Sleep Telemedicine Implementation Guide. Updated 2016. Available at: https://aasm.org/download-the-sleep-telemedicine-implementation-guide-a-free-resource-from-aasm/. Accessed March 1, 2024.
8. Singh J, Badr MS, Diebert W, et al. American Academy of Sleep Medicine (AASM) position paper for the use of telemedicine for the diagnosis and treatment of sleep disorders. *J Clin Sleep Med*. 2015; 11(10):1187-1198.
9. Interstate Medical Licensure Compact. Updated January 2021. Available at: https://www.imlcc.org. Accessed March 1, 2024.
10. Abbasi-Feinberg F. Telemedicine coding and reimbursement—current and future trends. *Sleep Med Clin*. 2020;15(3):417-429.
11. Fields BG. Regulatory, legal, and ethical considerations of telemedicine. *Sleep Med Clin*. 2020;15(3): 409-416.

12. American College of Physicians. Is Telehealth Ready for Prime Time? Updated January 2019. Available at: https://acpinternist.org/archives/2019/01/is-telehealth-ready-for-prime-time.htm. Accessed March 1, 2024.
13. Centers for Medicare and Medicaid Services. Health Care Provider Fact Sheet. Updated March 17, 2020. Available at: https://www.cms.gov/newsroom/fact-sheets/medicare-telemedicine-health-care-provider-fact-sheet. Accessed March 1, 2024.
14. American Academy of Sleep Medicine. Telemedicine. Updated January 2021. Available at: https://www.aasm.org/clinical-resources/telemedicine/. Accessed March 1, 2024.
15. Center for Connected Health Policy. Updated March 2021. Available at: https://www.cchpca.org/. Accessed March 1, 2024.
16. American Telemedicine Association. Updated March 2021. Available at: https://www.americantelemed.org/. Accessed March 1, 2024.
17. Health Resources and Services Administration. Federal Office of Rural Health Policy. Updated January 2021. Available at: https://www.hrsa.gov/rural-health/index.html. Accessed March 1, 2024.
18. Rural Information Hub. Rural Telehealth Toolkit. Updated January 2021. Available at: https://www.ruralhealthinfo.org/toolkits/telehealth/. Accessed March 1, 2024.
19. National Health Service. Technology Enabled Care Services (TECS). Updated 2020. Available at: https://www.england.nhs.uk/tecs/. Accessed March 1, 2024.
20. Venkateshiah SB, Hoque R, Collop N. Legal aspects of sleep medicine in the 21st century. *Chest*. 2018; 154(3):691-698.
21. Federation of State Medical Boards. States Waiving Licensure Requirements for Telehealth in Response to Covid-19. Updated March 16, 2021. Available at: https://www.fsmb.org/siteassets/advocacy/pdf/states-waiving-licensure-requirements-for-telehealth-in-response-to-covid-19.pdf. Accessed March 1, 2024.
22. National Council of State Boards of Nursing. Nurse Licensure Compact. Updated 2020. Available at: https://www.ncsbn.org/nurse-licensure-compact.htm. Accessed March 1, 2024.
23. Centers for Connected Health Policy. Credentialling and Privileging. Updated 2020. Available at: https://www.cchpca.org/telehealth-policy/credentialing-and-privileging. Accessed March 1, 2024.
24. U.S. Department of Health and Human Services. HIPAA for Professionals. Updated 2021. Available at: https://www.hhs.gov/hipaa/for-professionals/index.html. Accessed March 1, 2024.
25. HIPAAnswers. What Is HIPAA Compliant Telemedicine? Updated 2017. Available at: https://www.hipaanswers.com/what-is-hipaa-compliant-telemedicine. Accessed March 1, 2024.
26. U.S. Department of Health and Human Services. FAQs on Telehealth and HIPAA During the CO-VID-19 Nationwide Public Health Emergency. Updated 2020. Available at: https://www.hhs.gov/sites/default/files/telehealth-faqs-508.pdf. Accessed March 1, 2024.
27. Center for Connected Health Policy. HIPAA and Telehealth. Updated 2020. Available at: https://www.cchpca.org/sites/default/files/2018-09/HIPAA%20and%20Telehealth.pdf. Accessed March 1, 2024.
28. Center for Connected Health Policy. Current State Laws and Reimbursement Policies. Updated 2020. Available at: https://www.cchpca.org/telehealth-policy/current-state-laws-and-reimbursement-policies#. Accessed March 1, 2024.
29. Schutte-Rodin S. Telehealth, telemedicine, and obstructive sleep apnea. *Sleep Med Clin*. 2020;15(3):359-375.
30. Becker CD, Dandy K, Gaujean M, Fusaro M, Scurlock C. Legal perspectives on telemedicine part 1: legal and regulatory issues. *Perm J*. 2019;23:18-293.
31. U.S. Congress. Ryan Haight Online Pharmacy Consumer Protection Act. Updated 2008. Available at: https://www.congress.gov/bill/110th-congress/house-bill/6353/text. Accessed March 1, 2024.
32. Drug Enforcement Administration. DEA State Reciprocity. Updated 2020. Available at: https://www.deadiversion.usdoj.gov/GDP/(DEA-DC-018)(DEA067)%20DEA%20state%20reciprocity%20(final)(Signed).pdf. Accessed March 1, 2024.
33. Agency for Healthcare Research and Quality. AHRQ's Easy-to-Understand Telehealth Consent Form. Updated 2020. Available at: https://www.ahrq.gov/health-literacy/improve/informed-consent/index.html. Accessed March 1, 2024.
34. Brous E. Legal considerations in telehealth and telemedicine. *Am J Nurs*. 2016;116(9):64-67.
35. Bruhn HK. Telemedicine: dos and don'ts to mitigate liability risk. *J AAPOS*. 2020;24(4):195-196.
36. American Medical Association. Federal Stark Law Waivers During Covid-19. Updated December 7, 2020. Available at: https://www.ama-assn.org/system/files/2020-12/stark-waiver-guide.pdf. Accessed March 1, 2024.

37. Centers for Medicare and Medicaid Services. CMS Announces Historic Changes to Physician Self-Referral Regulations. Updated November 20, 2020. Available at: https://www.cms.gov/newsroom/press-releases/cms-announces-historic-changes-physician-self-referral-regulations. Accessed March 1, 2024.
38. Hayden EM, Erler KS, Fleming D. Telehealth ethics: the role of care partners. *Telemed J E Health.* 2020;26(8):976-977.
39. Aurora RN, Collop NA, Jacobowitz O, Thomas SM, Quan SF, Aronsky AJ. Quality measures for the care of adult patients with obstructive sleep apnea. *J Clin Sleep Med.* 2015;11(3):357-383.
40. American Medical Association. Ethical Practice in Telemedicine. Updated 2020. Available at: https://www.ama-assn.org/delivering-care/ethics/ethical-practice-telemedicine. Accessed March 1, 2024.
41. Watson NF, Rosen IM, Chervin RD, Board of Directors of the American Academy of Sleep M. The past is prologue: the future of sleep medicine. *J Clin Sleep Med.* 2017;13(1):127-135.
42. Katzow MW, Steinway C, Jan S. Telemedicine and health disparities during COVID-19. *Pediatrics.* 2020;146(2):e20201586.
43. Wall Street Journal Editorial Board. The Doctor Will Zoom You Now. Updated April 26, 2020. Available at: https://www.wsj.com/articles/the-doctor-will-zoom-you-now-11587935588. Accessed March 1, 2024.

CHAPTER 4

Coding and Reimbursement

Arveity R. Setty ■ Charles J. Bae

Telemedicine describes the practice of medicine using technology at a distance to deliver similar health care as if it was in the clinic. Telemedicine has been utilized in limited amounts for quite some time, but it has tremendously increased in the past 2½ years during the COVID-19 pandemic and public health emergency declaration. This has brought a lot of changes in the practice of remote medicine, and insurances have been covering more than before. The Centers for Medicare and Medicaid services (CMS) broadened access to care by allowing broad use of telemedicine services for a temporary duration and on an emergency basis under 1135 waiver authority and the Coronavirus Preparedness and Response Supplemental Appropriations Act.[1] The CMS and White House Task Forces wanted to ensure that US citizens have easy remote access to their providers, particularly those who are at high risk for complications from the coronavirus, in addition to helping contain the virus spread. Under this new waiver, Medicare not only paid for office visits, but also hospitalizations, and widened the place of service to a patient's home. A wide range of providers (e.g., doctors, nurse practitioners, licensed social workers, and psychologists) would all be able to offer telehealth to their patients. Prior to the pandemic, Medicare would only pay for telehealth on a limited basis.

Even before this waiver, the CMS was already making certain changes to their telemedicine coverage such as Virtual Check-Ins and E-visits. Once the public health emergency (PHE) is over, some of the relaxed billing practices might be terminated. But due to improvements in technology and Health Insurance Portability and Accountability Act of 1996 (HIPAA) policies in place, we expect that telemedicine will continue to be a covered service. An update on public health emergency and telemedicine is discussed later in this chapter.

Terminologies Used in Telemedicine

Telemedicine (synchronous): Services are live with interactive audio and visual transmissions of a physician-patient encounter from one site to another using telecommunication technology.

Telemedicine (asynchronous): Medical information is stored and forwarded to be reviewed by a physician or health care practitioner at a distant site. The medical information is reviewed without the patient being present. This is also referred to as *store-and-forward telehealth* or *non-interactive telecommunication.*

Originating site: Location where the patient is located.

Distant site: Location where the provider is located.

Who can perform telemedicine services and bill: A qualified health care professional (QHP) is an individual who is qualified by education, training, licensure/regulation, and facility privileging; performs a professional service within their scope of practice; and reports that professional service.

The Medicare definitions for a QHP are as follows:

■ Physician

■ Nurse practitioner

- Physician assistant
- Nurse midwife
- Clinical nurse specialist
- Certified registered nurse anesthetist
- Clinical psychologist and sociologist
- Registered dietician or nutrition professional

The Medicare definitions for an originating site are as follows:
- Office of the physician or practitioner
- Hospital (inpatient or outpatient)
- Critical access hospital
- Rural health clinic
- Federally qualified health center
- Hospital-based or critical access hospital-based renal dialysis center (including its satellites)
- Skilled nursing facility (SNF)
- Community mental health center
- Renal dialysis facility
- Homes of a beneficiary with end-stage renal disease (ESRD) receiving home dialysis
- Mobile stroke unit

Originating centers can charge a service fee by using the code Q3014. The originating site must be a rural, health professional shortage area (HPSA) or a non–metropolitan statistical area (MSA). This billing requirement has been relaxed during the COVID-19 PHE and has been extended until the end of 2024, and it is not clear how long it will be continued. The patient must be present during the visit and interactive audio and video telecommunications must be used, permitting real-time communication between the distant site and health care professional.

Current Procedural Terminology and the Healthcare Common Procedure Coding System

Current procedural terminology (CPT) codes are designated by the American Medical Association (AMA), and Healthcare Common Procedure Coding System (HCPCS) codes are designated by the CMS.

There are two levels of HCPCS[2]:

Level I of the HCPCS is composed of Current Procedural Terminology (CPT-4), a numeric coding system maintained by the AMA. The CPT-4 is a uniform coding system consisting of descriptive terms and identifying codes that are used primarily to identify medical services and procedures furnished by physicians and other health care professionals. These health care professionals use the CPT-4 to identify services and procedures for which they bill public or private health insurance programs. Level I of the HCPCS, the CPT-4 codes, does not include medical items or services that are regularly billed by suppliers other than physicians, thus level II was created.

Level II of the HCPCS is a standardized coding system that is used primarily to identify products, supplies, and services not included in the CPT-4 codes, such as ambulance services, durable medical equipment, prosthetics, orthotics, and supplies (DMEPOS) when used outside a physician's office. Because Medicare and other insurers cover a variety of services, supplies, and equipment that are not identified by CPT-4 codes, the level II HCPCS codes were established for submitting claims for these items.

There are also HCPCS level II codes that describe telemedicine services in the code descriptions.

HCPCS LEVEL II TELEHEALTH CODES

Type of Service

G0406-G0408 Follow-up Inpatient Consultation via Telehealth
G0425-G0427 Telehealth Consultation, Emergency Department
G0508, G0509 Telehealth Consultation, Critical Care

There are also certain G codes that are specifically used in sleep medicine to report a home sleep apnea test (G0398, G0399, and G0400). These have been in use since 2008. Most insurance companies accept G codes, but some require CPT codes like 95800, 95801, or 95806. An home sleep apnea test (HSAT) provider will need to contact each insurer they work with to identify which codes can be reported.

Modifiers for Telemedicine Coding

Since telemedicine started, there was a need for modifiers that could be used when the delivered service was not in person.

PLACE OF SERVICE CODE FOR TELEMEDICINE

Since telemedicine involves connecting to patient remotely, it is important to document the place of the service. The CMS introduced the Place of Service (POS) code 02 to identify the service as telemedicine. Code 02 indicates "the location where health services and health related services are provided or received, through telecommunication technology." It certifies that the service meets all telehealth requirements. Private payers have begun requiring this code as well.

GT/GQ MODIFIERS

A GT modifier indicates that the service was synchronous via interactive audio and video telecommunications. This is allowed only for institutional claims billed under critical access hospital (CAH) method II because they do not use POS codes. Some hospitals only require a GT modifier. Usually, it will mask when a payor does not need this to be reported and will change automatically to code 02 POS when a particular provider needs it for a claim process. A GQ modifier indicates that the service delivery was asynchronous.

MODIFIER 95

This indicates that the service was a real-time interactive audio and video interaction. In 2017, this was first described, but the updated 2020 CPT manual also includes Appendix P, which lists a summary of CPT codes that may be used for reporting synchronous (real-time) telemedicine services when appended by modifier 95. Some notable code families included in the list are:

Video-conferenced critical care services codes (0188T and 0189T), health and behavior assessment codes (96150 to 96154), and education and training for patient self-management codes (98960 to 98962). The last category might be useful in sleep medicine with PAP management.

CPT codes: In addition to Appendix P codes, the 2017 CPT Manual includes several codes that include telemedicine services in the code descriptions, with some examples here.

CPT TELEMEDICINE CODES TYPE OF SERVICE

99444 Online Evaluation and Management Service
99946-99448 Interprofessional Telephone/Internet Consultation

Evaluation and Management Codes

Sleep physicians also use Evaluation and Management (E/M) codes to bill for office visits. Medicare has an Evaluation and Management Services guide available with more details.[3] Evaluation and management codes are restricted to physicians and other qualified advanced nurse practitioners (e.g., NPs, PAs).

CPT CODE

99201 to 99205 New patient office visit with levels 1 to 5, respectively
99212 to 99215 Established patient office visit with levels 1 to 5, respectively

Whether it is a direct face-to-face evaluation or telemedicine encounter, the billing and reimbursement usually does not differ. A provider can bill either using medical decision making (MDM) requirements or based on time. The following table shows the new changes effective since 2021. When time is used, the provider can count all of the time spent on a particular patient on the same day of the encounter:
- Reviewing pertinent tests in preparation to see the patient
- Providing counseling and education for the patient/family/caregiver
- Ordering a medication, test, or procedure
- Documenting the medical record
- Obtaining and reviewing separately obtained history

This is a significant change since 2020, when one could only bill for the time spent with the patient (and over half of the time must have been spent counseling), or one had to make sure that MDM requirements were met in the office note.

IMPORTANT CODING CHANGES FROM JANUARY 2021[4]

On November 1, 2019, the CMS approved the Medicare physician fee schedule for 2020, which was to be effective starting January 1, 2021, and because they will affect how physicians code for telemedicine E/M visits as well, the codes will be reviewed and are as given in https://www.ama-assn.org/system/files/2023-e-m-descriptors-guidelines.pdf Accessed January 30, 2024.

Summary of Changes

Eliminate history and physical as elements for code selection. Providers must perform a medically appropriate history and/or physical examination, which will contribute to the total time (TT) spent with the patient as well as the medical decision making (MDM).

1. Documentation can be based on either MDM or TT, as noted in the table.
2. CPT code 99201 will be deleted, leaving four levels of new patient E/M codes but continuing with five levels of coding for established patients.
3. New add-on code for extended office visit time CPT code 99XXX and a new complexity add-on code GPC1X.
4. There are also some terminology contrasted for familiar language as follows:
   "Number of Diagnoses or Management Options" was changed to "Number and Complexity of Problems Addressed."

"Amount and/or Complexity of Data to be Reviewed" was changed to "Amount and/or Complexity of Data to be Reviewed and Analyzed."

"Risk of Complications and/or Morbidity or Mortality" was changed to "Risk of Complications and/or Morbidity or Mortality of Patient Management."

Coding for Telemedicine services is similar to coding for in-person clinic visits. For example, if a provider evaluates a follow-up patient for insomnia as a level 4 coding, the code would be 99214. But if the same service is performed via telehealth, the provider would submit the appropriate telemedicine modifier, and the code would be 99214-GT. Also, the originating site would bill for the facility fees for hosting the patient with HCPCS code Q3014.

To Qualify for a Particular Level of Service Based on MDM, two of the three Elements for That Level Need to be Met or Exceeded

Level of service (LOS) can also be chosen based on time, which is also shown here.

Other important CMS changes that were adopted from 2021 include increased value for the same E/M codes. The following are the changes in the relative value units (RVU) factor from 2020 to 2021.[5]

E/M Code	2020 Physician wRVU	2021 Physician wRVU	2022 Physician wRVU
99202	0.93	0.93	0.93
99203	1.42	1.60	1.60
99204	2.43	2.60	2.60
99205	3.17	3.50	3.50
99211	0.18	0.18	0.18
99212	0.48	0.70	0.70
99213	0.97	1.30	1.30
99214	1.50	1.92	1.92
99215	2.11	2.80	2.80

Non–Face-to-Face Services

Telehealth services without video are considered non–face-to-face telehealth services. Medicare recently started recognizing these communications as technology-based services.[1]

E-VISITS: ONLINE DIGITAL EVALUATION AND MANAGEMENT SERVICES

These are new additions to CPT as new digital communications tools (e.g., patient portals) started to be used. These allow health care professionals to efficiently connect with patients at home or any location and exchange information without going to doctor's office. To bill for these services, these communications must be initiated by the patient and are asynchronous. Consent is necessary on an annual basis, and this could be in the form of verbal consent. These communications can occur over a 7-day period. However, Medicare coinsurance and deductible would apply similar to any other health care service. Medicare part B also covers E-visits. There is no limit with respect to geographic area (not just rural).

---

*All levels require documentation of **chief complaint** (sign/symptom, ICD-10-CM diagnosis) and medically appropriate history and physical examination determined by the care team (does not contribute to LOS).

Physicians and nurse practitioners can bill the following codes:
- 99421: Online digital evaluation and management service, for an established patient, for up to 7 days, cumulative time during the 7 days; 5 to 10 minutes
- 99422: Online digital evaluation and management service, for an established patient, for up to 7 days cumulative time during the 7 days; 11 to 20 minutes
- 99423: Online digital evaluation and management service, for an established patient, for up to 7 days, cumulative time during the 7 days; 21 or more minutes

Clinicians who may not independently bill for evaluation and management visits, such as physical therapists, occupational therapists, speech language pathologists, and clinical psychologists (in sleep medicine this may apply for behavioral therapists who help children with behavioral insomnia), can also provide these E-visits and bill the following codes:
- G2061: Qualified non-physician health care professional online assessment and management, for an established patient, for up to seven days, cumulative time during the 7 days; 5 to 10 minutes
- G2062: Qualified non-physician health care professional online assessment and management service, for an established patient, for up to seven days, cumulative time during the 7 days; 11 to 20 minutes
- G2063: Qualified non-physician qualified health care professional assessment and management service, for an established patient, for up to seven days, cumulative time during the 7 days; 21 or more minutes.

Virtual Check-Ins: Brief Communication Technology-Based Service

Established Medicare patients in their home may have a brief communication service with practitioners via a number of communication technology modalities including a synchronous discussion over a telephone or exchange of information through video or image. These are supposed to be initiated by the patient; however, practitioners and sleep centers may need to educate patients on the availability of this service prior to patient initiation. Just like E-visits, these check-ins are expected to avoid unnecessary trips to doctor's office. These check-ins are for established patients and must not be related to a medical visit within the previous 7 days and do not lead to a medical visit within the next 24 hours (or sooner appointment if available). Patient consent is necessary (including verbal consent) for appropriate billing. Virtual check-ins can be conducted with a broader range of communication methods like telephone calls, unlike Medicare telehealth visits, which require audio and visual capabilities for real-time communication.

Physicians or other QHPs can bill using the following codes:
- HCPCS code G2012: Brief communication technology-based service (e.g., virtual check-in) by a physician or other qualified health care professional who can report evaluation and management services, provided to an established patient, not originating from a related E/M service provided within the previous 7 days or leading to an E/M service or procedure within the next 24 hours or soonest available appointment; 5 to 10 minutes of medical discussion.
- HCPCS code G2010: Remote evaluation of recorded video and/or images submitted by an established patient (e.g., store and forward), including interpretation with follow-up with the patient within 24 business hours, not originating from a related E/M service provided within the previous 7 days or leading to an E/M service or procedure within the next 24 hours or soonest available appointment (Table 4.1).

TABLE 4.1 ■ Difference Between Different Modalities of Telehealth Services Including Billing Codes. Obtained From CMS Website[1]

Type of Service	What Is the Service?	HCPCS/CPT Code	Patient Relationship With Provider
Medicare Telehealth Visit	A visit with a provider that uses telecommunication systems between the provider and patient	Common telehealth services include: 99201-99215 (Office or other outpatient visits) G0425-G0427 (Telehealth consultations, emergency department, or initial inpatient) G0406-G0408 (Follow-up inpatient telehealth consultations furnished to beneficiaries in hospitals or SNFs)	For new* or established patients
Virtual Check-In	A brief (5–10 minutes) check-in with a practitioner via telephone or other telecommunications device to decide whether an office visit or other service is needed A remote evaluation of recorded video and/or images submitted by an established patient	• HCPCS code G2012 • HCPCS code G2010	For established patients
E-Visit	A communication between a patient and provider through an online patient portal	99421 99422 99423 G2061 G2062 G2063	For established patients

*To the extent the 1135 waiver requires an established relationship. HHS will not conduct audits to ensure that such a prior relationship existed for claims submitted during this public health emergency.

Telephone Services

CMS has authorized the use of CPT codes 99441 to 99443 for telephone evaluation and management service by a physician or other qualified health care professional, who may report evaluation and management services provided to an established patient, parent, or guardian not originating from a related E/M service provided within the previous 7 days or leading to an E/M service or procedure within the next 24 hours or soonest available appointment.

Remote Physiologic Monitoring Services (CMS), Also Known as Remote Patient Monitoring (Digitally Stored Data Services)

In response to the increased delivery of telemedicine and remote monitoring services in a faster pace during the COVID-19 PHE, the CMS has deemed these to be reimbursable services.[6,7] These codes have been in existence for a few years, but CMS clarified in the CY 2021 Physician Fee Schedule (PFS) final rule the payment policies related to the RPM services described by CPT codes 99453, 99454, 99091, 99457, and 99458.

99453: This is a one-time practice expense reimbursing for the setup and patient education on RPM equipment. This code covers the initial setup of devices, training and education on the use of monitoring equipment, and any services needed to enroll the patient on-site. It needs 16 days of data within 30 days.

99454: This covers the supply and provisioning of devices used for RPM programs, and the code is billable only once in a 30-day billing period. Specifically, this code covers the costs associated with the leasing of a home-use medical device or devices to and for the patient.

99091: Although there is no exact code for PAP download and its assessment and monitoring of patients with sleep apnea remotely, 99091 generally suits well for the RPM coding for sleep services. CPT code 99091 is the collection and interpretation of physiologic data such as ECG, blood pressure, and glucose monitoring digitally stored and/or transmitted by the patient and/or caregiver to the physician or other qualified health care professional. The code requires a minimum of 30 minutes of interpretation and review and is billable once in a 30-day billing period. In this instance, the patient must have previously been seen in the clinic in person or by a telemedicine visit. In other words, these are established patients. There are no set number of conditions reported to qualify for this code. CPT code 99091 requires consent from patients, which can be obtained during the initial visit and must be documented in the patient's record.

99457 and 99458: These need a synchronous two-way communication.

Interprofessional Consultation

CPT codes 99446 to 99449 were first created in 2014 to capture the time spent by a consultant who is not in direct contact with the patient at the time of service. *Interprofessional consultation* (ITC) is defined as an assessment and management service in which a treating physician (e.g., primary care provider, hospital attending physician, or any QHP) requests the opinion and/or treatment advice of a consultant with specific specialty expertise to assist in the diagnosis and/or management of a patient's problem without the need for the patient's face-to-face interaction with the consultant.[8] These codes are typically used when a new problem arises or if a chronic issue is not well managed or worsens. Only a consultant can report these codes, and they require a verbal and written follow-up report.

The two ITC codes developed by the AMA Digital Medicine Payment Advisory Group are as follows:

- 99451 is reported by the consultant, allowing them to access data/information through the electronic health record (EHR) in addition to the telephone or Internet.
- 99452 is reported by the requesting/treating physician/QHP (e.g., the primary care physician).

Key Take Away Points

Consultant codes 99446 to 99449 and 99451:

- Can be reported for new or established patients and a new or exacerbated problem. Cannot be reported more than once per 7 days for the same patient and is cumulative time spent. You cannot report them if a transfer of care for a face-to-face consult within the next 14 days. A verbal consent must be documents in the patient medical record.

Requesting/treating physician/QHP code 99452:

- Is reported by the physician/QHP who is treating the patient and requesting the non–face-to-face consult for medical advice or opinion—and not for a transfer of care or a face-to-face consult. Patient must be under care of a physician/QHP at the time of consult and cannot be reported more than once per 14 days per patient. This also includes time preparing for the referral and/or communicating with the consultant Details of coding for Telehealth Visits, Online Digital Visits, Remote Patient Monitoring, and Telephone Evaluation and Management Services are available at https://www.ama-assn.org/practice-management/digital/ama-telehealth-policy-coding-payment.

Insurances and Payors

Almost all states offer telemedicine services for patients with **Medicare.** Contrary to **Medicaid,** which is State funded, Medicare is mostly state (although it is federal and state joint) managed and has traditionally been restrictive in their telehealth coverage. All 50 states and the District of Columbia reimburse for live video visits, but only 14 states with Medicaid programs reimburse for asynchronous "store and forward" technology. Only 19 states explicitly permit the patient's home to serve as the originating site. This has been relaxed during COVID-19 PHE, and it is not clear what will happen when the PHE ends.[9]

Commercial payers usually follow Medicare and Medicaid guidelines with respect to their reimbursement, and coverage can change from state to state. As long as state coverage and payment regulations are followed, individual commercial carriers have significant leeway to determine their own telehealth guidelines. Forty states and the District of Columbia currently passed laws that regulate private payer telehealth reimbursement. The major commercial carriers have published policies that give general guidance for which telehealth services are considered covered benefits.

Coverage for live video visits for established patients has been included as a covered benefit under all of the top five commercial payers, using CPT codes 99211-5 (limited to 99213-5 for some Blue Cross plans), place of service "02," and modifier -95 (or alternatively modifier—GT for Aetna, Blue Cross, and Cigna). However, prior to the expansion of telehealth coverage during the COVID-19 PHE, only one commercial payer (United Healthcare) had provisions for new patients to receive an evaluation via telemedicine. In this case, CPT 99499 was to be billed using place of service "02" instead of the usual new patient E/M code.

Coverage for non-video and asynchronous services has not been ubiquitous. Virtual check-in (G2012) has been covered by Aetna, Cigna, Humana, and United Healthcare, but not by all Blue Cross plans. United Healthcare, on the other hand, has only covered remote evaluation of recorded video/image (CPT G2010). Aetna and Blue Cross have covered telephone visits (CPT 99441-3,

98966-8) for commercial plan members and by Humana for its Medicare Advantage members only (99441-3). Humana's Medicare Advantage members have also been some of the only commercial insurance beneficiaries with coverage for E-visits (CPT 99421-3). These coverages will keep changing with time, and policies should be reviewed on an ongoing basis.

Direct-to-consumer (DtC) is where a consumer directly can access other health care providers, especially when their own physicians do not offer telehealth services. When given the choice, most patients prefer to receive telehealth from their existing health care providers.[9] These services are generally self-pay because they typically are not a covered insurance benefit. Patients might choose to pay out of pocket to utilize telehealth services due to convenience, easy accessibility, and immediacy of receiving care.

Irrespective of the insurance or payment differences, state licensing rules for telemedicine must be met. However, during the PHE, state boundaries related to licensure were removed by most states. Some states have reinstated licensure restrictions, and this will continue to change and must be followed closely to provide telehealth services legally.

Billing Without the Patient During Telemedicine

It is expected that the patient or caregiver is present during the telemedicine services to be billed. As a pediatric sleep physician, it is common for practitioners to see a parent only during a follow-up visit. If there is an established relationship with the child and caregiver, this is not a big concern because the care plan is always discussed with the parent or caregiver. This happens routinely during in-person visits. However, for an initial consult, the child should be present during the visit. There are other scenarios when the patient may not be present during a follow-up visit, such as when the patient cannot communicate due to medical problems.

Billing Outside State Borders

It is very important to make sure and be aware of the state licensing requirements for telemedicine. To bill for the visit, the patient must be within the state where the provider is licensed. This requirement has been relaxed during COVID-19 PHE but will change back once PHE ends. If state licensing requirements are not met, it is inappropriate to bill those visits. Practitioners can use this link for up-to-date state rules and licensing requirements: https://www.fsmb.org/siteassets/advocacy/pdf/states-waiving-licensure-requirements-for-telehealth-in-response-to-covid-19.pdf. This can serve as an updated resource for COVID-19 PHE and state licensing requirements.

Telehealth Policy Changes After the Covid-19 Public Health Emergency

The PHE will be ending shortly, but most of the telemedicine services will be continued until December 31, 2024. Medicare changes through the PHE and afterward are described on their website.[9]

PERMANENT MEDICARE CHANGES

- Federally Qualified Health Centers (FQHCs) and Rural Health Clinics (RHCs) can serve as a distant site provider for behavioral/mental telehealth services.
- Medicare patients can receive telehealth services for behavioral/mental health care in their home.
- There are no geographic restrictions for originating site for behavioral/mental telehealth services.

- Behavioral/mental telehealth services can be delivered using audio-only communication platforms.
- Rural hospital emergency departments are accepted as an originating site.

TEMPORARY MEDICARE CHANGES THROUGH DECEMBER 31, 2024

- A Federally Qualified Health Center (FQHC)/Rural Health Clinic (RHC) can serve as a distant site provider for non-behavioral/mental telehealth services.
- Medicare patients can receive telehealth services authorized in the Calendar Year 2023 Medicare Physician Fee Schedule in their home.
- There are no geographic restrictions for originating site for non-behavioral/mental telehealth services.
- Some non-behavioral/mental telehealth services can be delivered using audio-only communication platforms.
- An in-person visit within 6 months of an initial behavioral/mental telehealth service, and annually thereafter, is not required.
- Telehealth services can be provided by a physical therapist, occupational therapist, speech language pathologist, or audiologist.

TEMPORARY CHANGES THROUGH THE END OF THE COVID-19 PUBLIC HEALTH EMERGENCY

- Telehealth can be provided as an excepted benefit.
- Medicare-covered providers may use any non-public facing application to communicate with patients without risking any federal penalties—even if the application is not in compliance with HIPAA.

Conclusion

The COVID-19 PHE has pushed the adoption and utilization of telemedicine to levels that were not seen pre-pandemic. Reasons for the accelerated use of telemedicine included access to care in a safe manner, relaxation of state licensure restrictions to practice across state lines, and continued reimbursement for services. During the COVID-19 PHE, changes to coding for E/M services were introduced in January 2021 as well. Telemedicine is an important tool to provide patient care, but close attention must be paid to the continuously changing rules and regulations.

Additional Resources

Complete List of CME Telehealth Services. Available at: https://www.cms.gov/Medicare/Medicare-General-Information/Telehealth/Telehealth-Codes. Accessed March 1, 2024.

General Provider Telehealth and Telemedicine Toolkit. Available at: https://www.cms.gov/files/document/general-telemedicine-toolkit.pdf. Accessed March 1, 2024.

COVID-19 FAQ's on Medicare Fee-for-Service Billing. Available at: https://edit.cms.gov/files/document/medicare-telehealth-frequently-asked-questions-faqs-31720.pdf. Accessed March 1, 2024.

Medicare Telehealth Services. Available at: https://edit.cms.gov/files/document/medicare-telehealth-frequently-asked-questions-faqs-31720.pdf and detailed information at https://www.cms.gov/Medicare/Medicare-General-Information/Telehealth. Accessed March 1, 2024.

Medicare Telehealth payment Eligibility Analyzer. Available at: https://data.hrsa.gov/tools/medicare/telehealth. Accessed March 1, 2024.

References

1. Medicare Telemedicine Health Care Provider Fact Sheet. Available at: https://www.cms.gov/newsroom/fact-sheets/medicare-telemedicine-health-care-provider-fact-sheet. Accessed March 1, 2024.
2. HCPCS Coding Questions. Available at: https://www.cms.gov/Medicare/Coding/MedHCPCSGenInfo/HCPCS_Coding_Questions. Accessed March 1, 2024.
3. Telehealth Services Covered by Medicare and Included in CPT Code Set. https://www.ama-assn.org/system/files/2020-05/telehealth-services-covered-by-Medicare-and-included-in-CPT-code-set.pdf. Accessed March 1, 2024.
4. Abbasi-Feinberg F. Telemedicine coding and reimbursement—current and future trends. *Sleep Med Clin.* 2020;15(3):417-429.
5. E/M Codes RVU Factor for 2021. AASM website: https://aasm.org/evaluation-and-management-code-changes-for-2021. Accessed March 1, 2024.
6. Final Policy, Payment, and Quality Provisions Changes to the Medicare Physician Fee Schedule for Calendar Year 2021. Available at: https://www.cms.gov/newsroom/fact-sheets/final-policy-payment-and-quality-provisions-changes-medicare-physician-fee-schedule-calendar-year-1. Accessed March 1, 2024.
7. Your Guide to Reimbursement for Remote Patient Monitoring. Available at: https://www.validic.com/resources/detail/your-guide-to-reimbursement-for-remote-patient-monitoring. Accessed March 1, 2024.
8. Bajowala SS, Milosch J, Bansal C. Telemedicine pays: billing and coding update. *Curr Allergy Asthma Rep.* 2020;20(10):60.
9. Telehealth Policy Changes After the COVID-19 Public Health Emergency. Available at: https://telehealth.hhs.gov/providers/policy-changes-during-the-covid-19-public-health-emergency/policy-changes-after-the-covid-19-public-health-emergency. Accessed March 1, 2024.

CHAPTER 5

Sleep Telemedicine: Reimagining the Health Care Team

Janet Hilbert ■ Barry Fields

Sleep Medicine Care Delivery

BACKGROUND

Change is constant, and health care is no exception. The diagnosis-centered, prescriptive, physician-led care of the not-too-distant past has evolved into more patient-centered, collaborative, team-based care (Figure 5.1). In part, this change stemmed from work by the Picker Foundation ultimately leading to the principles of patient-centered care.[1] In 2001, the Institute of Medicine landmark report "Crossing the Quality Chasm" called for redesign of the U.S. health care system. Six specific aims for health care improvement were identified: (1) safety, (2) effectiveness, (3) equity, (4) timeliness, (5) patient-centeredness, and (6) efficiency.

The process has been slow, but the rate of change is accelerating.[2] Drivers of change include the digital health revolution, consumerism, unsustainable cost structures, workforce changes, and, most recently, coronavirus disease 2019 (COVID-19).[2,3]

THE PAST

The field of sleep medicine has evolved considerably over the years.[1,4,5] In the past, much of sleep medicine focused on a single diagnosis (obstructive sleep apnea [OSA]), using a single test performed at a centralized sleep center (polysomnography) interpreted by a sleep physician who prescribed limited treatment options (continuous positive airway pressure [CPAP] or surgery). Follow-up was limited to clinical reassessment and repeat polysomnography as needed. Similarly, diagnostic and treatment options of other sleep disorders were also limited.

THE PRESENT

Over time, this paradigm shifted.[1] With increased understanding of the pathophysiology of disease, options for diagnostic testing, more personalized treatments, and ability to monitor outcomes objectively, sleep medicine has become more patient-centered, more collaborative, and more focused on chronic disease management and long-term care (see Figure 5.1). Sleep laboratories of the past have transitioned to sleep centers where clinical care is provided by a multidisciplinary team of physicians and advanced practice professionals, nurses, respiratory therapists (RTs), sleep technologists, psychologists, and others.[6] This multidisciplinary team often interfaces with consultants in neurology, pulmonology, dentistry, cardiology, nutrition, metabolism, otorhinolaryngology, oral/maxillofacial surgery, and bariatric surgery.

Given the large number of individuals with sleep disorders and the relatively few board-certified sleep physicians, collaborative models of health care have been proposed.[4,7] The patient-centered medical home (PCMH) care model is a care delivery system in which care is coordinated by

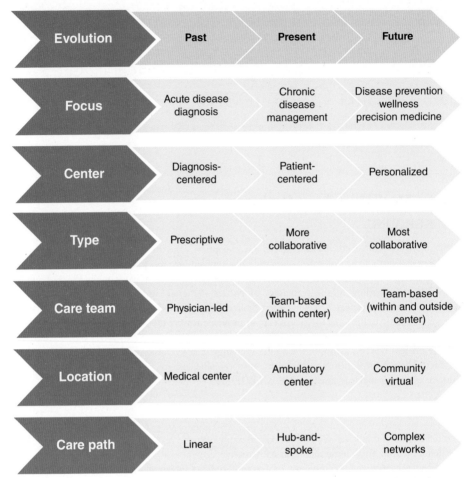

Evolution	Past	Present	Future
Focus	Acute disease diagnosis	Chronic disease management	Disease prevention wellness precision medicine
Center	Diagnosis-centered	Patient-centered	Personalized
Type	Prescriptive	More collaborative	Most collaborative
Care team	Physician-led	Team-based (within center)	Team-based (within and outside center)
Location	Medical center	Ambulatory center	Community virtual
Care path	Linear	Hub-and-spoke	Complex networks

Figure 5.1 Conceptual framework of the evolution of sleep medicine health care models over time.

primary care practitioners.[7] The American Academy of Sleep Medicine (AASM) Future of Sleep Medicine Task Force reviewed multiple health care delivery models for sleep specialists in 2010 and 2011 and concluded that sleep medicine is best described as a partner or "neighbor" in the care process.[7] In the "hub-and-spoke" collaborative model of care (with primary care practitioners as the spokes and the sleep center as the hub), primary care practitioners evaluate patients with suspected sleep disorders and then refer to the hub for further evaluation, testing, or complex management.[4] Coordinated care may include informal exchange, coordinated management, or comanagement. The success of such collaboration depends on the expertise of the primary care practitioners, clear delineation of responsibilities, and ongoing communication.

Several studies have demonstrated that primary care practitioners can manage straightforward OSA. However, lack of time, variable knowledge of sleep medicine, poor specialist access, and lack of clarity of roles are barriers to optimal OSA care.[8] Increased integration of primary care practitioners and more effective technology have been suggested as potential solutions. The "sustainable methods, algorithms, and research tools for delivering optimal care" (SMART DOCS) study is a longitudinal study commenced in 2013 comparing a novel out-patient care delivery model for sleep disorders with conventional care.[9] The central question is whether this new model improves care from a patient perspective and improves the health of patients while also controlling costs.

THE FUTURE

Looking toward the future, increased understanding of mechanisms of disease, technological advances, and the explosion of personalized data should lead to more personalized health care, focused not just on chronic disease management but also on disease prevention. The "predictive, preventive, personalized, and participatory" (P4) approach in medicine includes assessment of genomic, environmental, and phenotypic measurements to better diagnose and treat disease and maximize wellness.[10] Health care of the future (see Figure 5.1) will require multidisciplinary practitioners in complex networks working together to care for patients in the community. Increasing reliance on patient-provided data and decision-making enhanced by artificial intelligence (AI) and machine learning will add to the transformation of care.[2]

Impact of Sleep Telemedicine on the Health Care Team

DEFINITIONS

Telemedicine may be defined as clinical care provided remotely through telecommunication (Figure 5.2). It is part of the larger system of remote health care services that encompasses both clinical and non-clinical services (telehealth). Telemedicine may be delivered synchronously, with real-time interaction between patients and medical practitioners, or it may be delivered

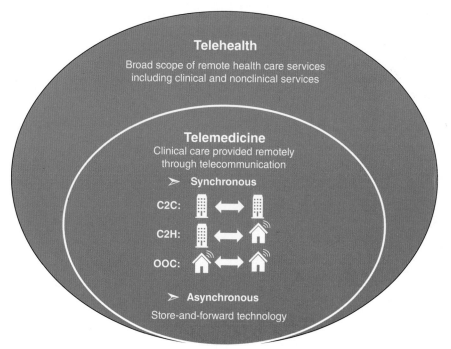

Figure 5.2 Relationship between telemedicine and telehealth. *C2C,* Center-to-center; *C2H,* center-to-home; *OOC,* out-of-center.

asynchronously through "store-and-forward" interaction. Asynchronous sleep telemedicine (such as cloud-based CPAP monitoring, remote interpretation of sleep studies, and electronic messaging) has been widely used for some time. Synchronous sleep telemedicine has historically been limited by federal and state regulations, but there has been exponential growth during the COVID-19 pandemic.[11,12] Synchronous telemedicine is characterized by the location of the patient (originating site) and location of the practitioner (distant site). Both the patient and practitioner may be at separate clinical centers (center-to-center [C2C]), the practitioner may be at a clinical center with the patient at home or at another nonclinical location (center-to-home [C2H]), or both the patient and practitioner may be at home or at other nonclinical locations (out-of-center [OOC]).

POTENTIAL ADVANTAGES AND CHALLENGES

In many ways, sleep medicine is a field ideally suited to telemedicine, which in turn has the potential to revolutionize the care of individuals with chronic diseases such as OSA, diabetes, and hypertension.[13] Comprehensive management of OSA by telemedicine (see Chapters 17-20) has been shown to be feasible in multiple studies.[14-16] Internet-delivered cognitive behavioral therapy (CBT-i) has been shown to be effective in insomnia (see Chapter XX).

Telemedicine allows the current practice of sleep medicine to move from the present into the future (see Figure 5.1). It can be viewed as part of a "virtual PCMH" that includes other telehealth strategies to improve access to care, support patient self-management, and improve care coordination.[17] Telemedicine has multiple potential advantages compared with in-person care, but there are also challenges, both for patients (Table 5.1) and for the sleep health care team (Table 5.2). In a qualitative study of tele-monitoring in primary care, practitioners raised concerns, many of which could be addressed by improved system design.[18] In a real-world description of the rapid adoption of telemedicine due to COVID-19, telemedicine was not an unqualified success. The authors cite several subthemes including the importance of accommodating patient choice, the need to match encounter type to the visit platform, the hazards of remote care, and the need to adapt advanced team-based care with in-room support to the virtual environment.[19]

TABLE 5.1 ■ Potential Advantages and Challenges of Sleep Telemedicine From the Patient Perspective

	In-Person Care	Telemedicine
Potential advantages	• Familiar • Close team member–patient relationships	• Convenient • Time-saving • Less expensive • Potential to decrease health disparities (e.g., no need for transportation) • Easier family participation • Improved medication reconciliation
Potential challenges	• Inconvenient • Time-consuming • More expensive (e.g., travel, parking, time off work) • Potential to increase health disparities (e.g., need for transportation)	• Need for technology hardware/software • Comfort with using technology • Potential to increase health disparities (e.g., need for technology)

TABLE 5.2 ■ Potential Advantages and Challenges of Sleep Telemedicine From the Health Care Team Perspective

	In-Person Model	Telemedicine
Potential advantages	• Close working relationships within center (e.g., team huddles)	• Improved working relationships throughout the system as a whole with virtual support • More efficient care
Potential challenges	• Fragmented working relationships between team members within the sleep center and outside center	• Not appropriate for certain symptoms or diagnoses • Limited capability for physical examination • Types of encounters and care roles subject to regulations • Need for intensive information technology support to be successful • Physical isolation of practitioners, need for within-center team support to be successful • Need for care coordination to be successful

EVOLVING ROLES OF SLEEP TEAM MEMBERS

The sleep team within the present-day sleep center includes many if not all of the following: board-certified sleep physicians; board-certified sleep psychologists; advanced practice providers (APPs) including nurse practitioners (NPs) and physician assistants (PAs); sleep technologists; nurses including registered nurses (RNs) and licensed practical nurses (LPNs); medical assistants; RTs; and support staff. In 2016, the AASM Task Force listed multiple recommendations for the use of telemedicine in sleep medicine.[11] Among these, those that relate to the health care team include the following:

- Clinical care services for telemedicine should mirror those of in-person care.
- Clinical judgment should be exercised when determining the scope and extent of telemedicine applications.
- Roles, expectations, and responsibilities of practitioners should be defined.
- Telemedicine should aim to promote a care model in which sleep specialists, patients, primary care providers, and other team members aim to improve the value of health care delivery in a coordinated fashion.

With telemedicine (and telehealth in general), new roles may emerge (e.g., tele-presenters in C2C visits, virtual care coordinators in complex models of care). Other roles become more important (e.g., information technology [IT]). Some roles may change (e.g., sleep technologists and RTs shifting to more patient education and follow-up and less data acquisition and scoring). Including the entire health care team (Figure 5.3) in decision-making is critical to the success of a telemedicine program.[20]

Health Care Team Member Roles Over the Sleep Medicine Care Continuum

Patients move through phases of sleep care from the initial suspicion of a sleep disorder through diagnosis, treatment, and follow-up. Along the way, there may be multiple branch points or detours. Patients may have more than one diagnosis. They may require additional support during treatment or may require alternative treatments. They may need advanced technologies for follow-up. Sleep health care team members (see Figure 5.3) may have varying roles and levels of involvement throughout this continuum, and a coordinated approach is essential.

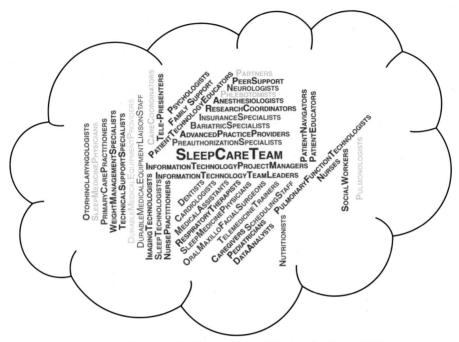

Figure 5.3 Word cloud depicting members of the sleep health care team.

PRIOR TO SLEEP EVALUATION

Many patients initially report symptoms to their primary care practitioners or other specialists, who subsequently refer for sleep consultation. However, given multiple barriers (e.g., little sleep education in medical school curricula, lack of time), sleep disorders often remain unrecognized and untreated.

Sleep center physicians and other sleep educators may offer educational programs to increase sleep knowledge regarding when to refer as well as how to potentially participate in long-term management.[18] Working with IT, sleep questionnaires and simple screens may be incorporated into the electronic medical record (EMR). In one study of individuals who completed sleep screening surveys, participants believed screening was valuable, and it often led to further treatment actions.[21] In a pilot project of sleep education for community practitioners, participants reported improved comfort in managing sleep complaints, but conflicts and lack of time were major participation barriers.[22]

As evidenced by the increase in consumer wearable and nearable sleep technology, individuals are increasingly interested in improving sleep.[23] This, in turn, may lead to more patient-initiated sleep evaluations.

INFORMATION TECHNOLOGY SUPPORT

For a telemedicine program to be successful, basic hardware and software requirements must be met, and privacy and security must be assured[20] (see Chapters 3 and 10). Interfacing with the EMR is ideal. Initial and ongoing education and support are critical for practitioners, staff, and patients. The IT team may include a team leader, project managers, data analysts, technical support specialists, telemedicine trainers, and patient technology educators.

ADMINISTRATIVE SUPPORT

Support for scheduling, pre-authorization, coding, billing, and other support functions must be in place for telemedicine, similar to in-person care. With IT support, there may be opportunities for patient self-scheduling and automatic text or EMR appointment reminders. This may free up staff to administer electronic questionnaires, triage patient messages via the EMR portal or traditional methods, or assume other roles (e.g., patient technology educators, telemedicine trainers).

SLEEP CLINICAL CARE

Per 2016 AASM recommendations, clinical care services for telemedicine should mirror those of in-person care.[11] For initial consultations, physicians and other trained practitioners should follow the same standards for history-taking and documentation as in-person care. Roles of APPs should be clearly defined and follow the scope of practice for their field and institution. Nursing and medical assistants may assist with questionnaires, elements of the history, medication reconciliation, and so forth, within their scope of practice. In C2C telemedicine visits, patient presenters may assist with the physical examination and other elements of the visit. Maintaining a team-based approach during the virtual visit will ideally reduce "distracted doctoring" and improve the patient and practitioner experience.[19]

For follow-up care, all of the aforementioned recommendations apply, with care mirroring in-person care. Prior studies have shown noninferiority of OSA care performed by trained nurses and RTs compared with sleep physician care.[24] Telemedicine care for OSA improves access and results in acceptable outcomes, but the roles of specific team members were not specified.[14-16] State, local, and federal regulations and insurance guidelines must be consulted for feasibility.

SLEEP TESTING

Attended, in-laboratory polysomnography is considered the "gold-standard" test in sleep medicine, and it was the primary test performed for many years. However, after the approval of home sleep apnea testing as a viable test for OSA, the field of sleep medicine changed with many centers closing or restructuring.[5] Sleep technologists pivoted to increase home sleep apnea testing, although polysomnography remains appropriate at the present time for complicated sleep-disordered breathing or non-OSA sleep disorders. For both polysomnography and home sleep apnea testing, AASM guidelines should be followed for data acquisition and scoring and for study interpretation[11] (see Chapters 16 and 17).

Polysomnography may be successfully performed in the home with remote monitoring.[25,26] Machine learning algorithms may improve polysomnography scoring.[27] Although traditional metrics of sleep-disordered breathing may be useful, other data in the polysomnography may ultimately prove to be helpful.[28] Newer technologies to define sleep-disordered breathing or assess sleep, including consumer sleep technologies, may make traditional sleep testing less important.[28,29]

RESEARCH COORDINATION

Telehealth has the potential to connect patients, clinicians, and researchers. The Patient-Centered Outcomes Research Institute (PCORI) was established to develop a network to foster patient-centered comparative effectiveness research. SMART DOCS is one example of a PCORI-sponsored study that compared a coordinated care management approach in sleep disorders with a conventional care approach.[9] Another PCORI-funded study examined the role of peer buddies in improving satisfaction among patients with OSA.[30]

CARE COORDINATION

With increasing complexity of care within and outside the sleep center, care coordinators may serve a vital role navigating patients through the phases of sleep care from screening through diagnosis, various active treatments, and follow-up. Patient navigators (who may be nurses, other members of the health care team, or nonmedical professionals) help patients successfully navigate complex health care systems in chronic disease such as cancer.[31] Sleep medicine care can be similarly complex; patient navigation may be useful but is as yet untested.

BEHAVIORAL SLEEP MEDICINE

With synchronous telemedicine, patients may meet with psychologists for individual or group CBTi. In asynchronous telemedicine, self-directed insomnia treatments may occur through web-based or mobile applications. Telemedicine-based CBTi has been shown to be noninferior to traditional CBTi[32-34] (see Chapter 15). Although actigraphy and sleep diaries are traditionally used in the management of insomnia and circadian rhythm disorders, consumer sleep technology may also provide objective, longitudinal sleep assessment to improve patient care.[23]

POSITIVE AIRWAY PRESSURE THERAPY MANAGEMENT

In a home-based approach to diagnosis and treatment of uncomplicated OSA, home sleep apnea testing is typically followed by auto-adjusting CPAP. Fine-tuning of therapy is based on clinical symptoms and assessment of CPAP device data. Data on remote CPAP titration (with a technical team remotely adjusting CPAP settings) are limited to a small pilot study.[25,35]

Assessment of CPAP device data is the standard of care in the management of OSA,[11] with data historically downloaded and reviewed with the patient at the time of an in-person visit. With current CPAP devices, remote patient monitoring is possible with real-time ability to modify and optimize therapy.[6] Data can now be reviewed during synchronous telemedicine visits through "screen-sharing technology" or may be reviewed asynchronously by the care team. The use of telemedicine approaches has been shown to improve CPAP adherence[36-40] (see Chapters 19 and 20). EHR integration of CPAP data is possible and may improve timeliness in detecting efficacy, adherence, or leak issues and thus improve patient care. Current barriers to implementation of CPAP-EHR integration include privacy issues and cost.[41]

MEDICATION MANAGEMENT

Data on telemedicine approaches to pharmacologic management of sleep disorders are lacking. The AASM does endorse the use of live interactive telemedicine for prescription of sedative hypnotics, stimulants, wakefulness-promoting medications, and other controlled substances prescribed by the sleep practitioner.[11] Medication prescribing via telemedicine is subject to local, state, and federal regulation (see Chapter 3). Medication reconciliation may be performed by nursing during synchronous or asynchronous encounters. Pharmacists may also have role in patient education, review of medication history, therapy management, and drug utilization.[42] Whether telemedicine medication review improves patient outcomes is the subject of future study.[43]

EDUCATION AND SUPPORT

Remote CPAP monitoring with telemedicine support by the sleep care team has been shown to improve CPAP adherence[40] (see Chapters XX and XX). Additionally, phone-based peer support has been found to improve satisfaction among patients with OSA.[30] In a current PCORI implementation project, a project team teaches sleep center staff, typically CPAP coordinators or nurse navigators, to train peers in the support program.[44]

SPECIALTY CARE COORDINATION

Electronic consultations (E-consults) are electronic, asynchronous, practitioner-to-practitioner consultations that rely on information provided within the EMR. E-consults may be directed to the sleep team (e.g., a nonsleep practitioner may ask for guidance as to whether a patient's symptoms warrant further evaluation). In the hub-and-spoke model of care in which a primary care practitioner is assuming comanagement, the practitioner may need an opinion as to whether CPAP data are acceptable. Effective communication is essential for the success of such a care model.[4,8]

Alternatively, sleep practitioners may seek E-consults from other specialists when the question is straightforward or may choose to refer for in-person or telemedicine consultations. Sleep medicine is multidisciplinary, and optimal care may require input from neurology, pulmonology, cardiology, otorhinolaryngology, dentistry, oral maxillofacial surgery, nutrition, bariatric surgery, and other specialists.

Interdisciplinary telemedicine including multiple health care professionals along with the patient is possible with many telemedicine platforms and may be a preferred option in some cases.[45] In a qualitative study of telemedicine from the palliative care literature, multidisciplinary telemedicine was found to facilitate direct cooperation among health care professionals.[46]

ANCILLARY TESTING

Additional testing may be required in certain clinical situations. For example, radiography, spirometry, echocardiography, pulmonary function testing, arterial blood gas testing, laboratory testing (e.g., measurements of serum bicarbonate, iron stores), home oximetry, and carbon dioxide monitoring are just some of the tests that may be appropriate in select patients seen in a comprehensive sleep center. Some noninvasive ventilators integrate oximetry and carbon dioxide monitoring into their platforms for remote monitoring.[47]

PERIPHERAL DEVICES AND CONSUMER SLEEP TECHNOLOGY

Electronic stethoscopes and other peripherals are currently being used by tele-presenters during C2C visits to assist with the physical examination.[11] Wearable devices, nearable devices, and mobile applications are increasingly being used by consumers to track measures of health and wellness including sleep[23,29] (see Chapter XX). Use of these technologies diagnostically is currently limited by siloed businesses, proprietary algorithms, lack of validation, and unknown generalizability. A collaborative effort among manufacturers, researchers, and clinicians will be needed to overcome these barriers.[23,29] Review of relevant consumer-tracked health outcomes (e.g., blood pressure, blood glucose, and measures of sleep tracked simultaneously) may ultimately prove useful in managing patients with sleep disorders longitudinally and in improving population sleep health.

CONCLUSION

Sleep medicine has evolved as a specialty. Team-based, collaborative care is the norm. Sleep telemedicine, starting with asynchronous store-and-forward technology and now with expanded synchronous clinical care, has the potential to dramatically improve patient care. Team-based telemedicine is not without its challenges, but these should be surmountable with education, experience, and innovative technology. There are increasing opportunities for members of the health care team to participate in care through all phases and there are more opportunities to expand the health care team. Looking toward the future, telemedicine will be part of the health care landscape that will allow personalized care focused not just on chronic disease management but also on optimizing sleep health.

References

1. Hilbert J, Yaggi HK. Patient-centered care in obstructive sleep apnea: a vision for the future. *Sleep Med Rev*. 2018;37:138-147.
2. Zimlichman E, Nicklin W, Aggrawal R, Bates DW. Health Care 2030: the coming transformation. *NEJM Catalyst*. 2021. https://catalyst.nejm.org/doi/full/10.1056/CAT.20.0569. Accessed March 27, 2021.
3. Hollander JE, Sites FD. The transition from reimagining to recreating healthcare is now. *NEJM Catalyst*. 2020. https://catalyst.nejm.org/doi/full/10.1056/CAT.20.0093. Accessed March 27, 2021.
4. Watson NF, Rosen IM, Chervin RD, Board of Directors of the American Academy of Sleep Medicine. The past is prologue: the future of sleep medicine. *J Clin Sleep Med*. 2017;13(1):127-135.
5. Kirsch DB. Disruption in health care (and sleep medicine): "It's the end of the world as we know it...and i feel fine." *J Clin Sleep Med*. 2019;15(9):1185-1188.
6. Shelgikar AV, Durmer JS, Joynt KE, et al. Multidisciplinary sleep centers: strategies to improve care of sleep disorders patients. *J Clin Sleep Med*. 2014;10(6):693-697.
7. Strollo PJ Jr, Badr MS, Coppola MP, et al. The future of sleep medicine. *Sleep*. 2011;34(12):1613-1619.
8. Pendharkar SR, Blades K, Kelly JE, et al. Perspectives on primary care management of obstructive sleep apnea: a qualitative study of patients and health care providers. *J Clin Sleep Med*. 2021;17(1):89-98.
9. Kushida CA, Nichols DA, Holmes TH, et al. SMART DOCS: a new patient-centered outcomes and coordinated-care management approach for the future practice of sleep medicine. *Sleep*. 2015;38(2):315-326.
10. Sagner M, McNeil A, Puska P, et al. The P4 health spectrum—A predictive, preventive, personalized and participatory continuum for promoting healthspan. *Prog Cardiovasc Dis*. 2017;59(5):506-521.
11. Singh J, Badr MS, Diebert W, et al. American Academy of Sleep Medicine (AASM) position paper for the use of telemedicine for the diagnosis and treatment of sleep disorders. *J Clin Sleep Med*. 2015;11(10):1187-1198.
12. Shamim-Uzzaman QA, Bae CJ, Ehsan Z, et al. The use of telemedicine for the diagnosis and treatment of sleep disorders: an American Academy of Sleep Medicine update. *J Clin Sleep Med*. 2021;17(5):1103-1107.
13. Corbett JA, Opladen JM, Bisognano JD. Telemedicine can revolutionize the treatment of chronic disease. *Int J Cardiol Hypertens*. 2020;7:100051.
14. Fields BG, Behari PP, McCloskey S, et al. Remote ambulatory management of veterans with obstructive sleep apnea. *Sleep*. 2016;39(3):501-509.
15. Lugo VM, Garmendia O, Suarez-Giron M, et al. Comprehensive management of obstructive sleep apnea by telemedicine: clinical improvement and cost-effectiveness of a Virtual Sleep Unit. A randomized controlled trial. *PLoS One*. 2019;14(10):e0224069.
16. Sarmiento KF, Folmer RL, Stepnowsky CJ, et al. National expansion of sleep telemedicine for Veterans: the TeleSleep Program. *J Clin Sleep Med*. 2019;15(9):1355-1364.
17. Nuss S, Camayd-Munoz C, Jonas R, et al. Defining the virtual patient-centered medical home. *Clin Pediatr (Phila)*. 2018;57(13):1592-1596.
18. Hanley J, Pinnock H, Paterson M, McKinstry B. Implementing telemonitoring in primary care: learning from a large qualitative dataset gathered during a series of studies. *BMC Fam Pract*. 2018;19(1):118.
19. Sinsky CA, Jerzak JT, Hopkins KD. Telemedicine and team-based care. *Mayo Clin Proc*. 2021;96(2):429-437.
20. Khosla S. Implementation of synchronous telemedicine into clinical practice. *Sleep Med Clin*. 2020;15(3):347-358.
21. Pascoe M, Alberts J, Wang L, et al. Feasibility of electronic sleep disorder screening in healthcare workers of a large healthcare system. *Sleep Med*. 2020;73:181-186.

22. Parsons EC, Mattox EA, Beste LA, et al. Development of a sleep telementorship program for rural department of Veterans Affairs primary care providers: sleep Veterans Affairs extension for community healthcare outcomes. *Ann Am Thorac Soc.* 2017;14(2):267-274.
23. Goldstein C. Current and future roles of consumer sleep technologies in sleep medicine. *Sleep Med Clin.* 2020;15(3):391-408.
24. Pendharkar SR, Tsai WH, Penz ED, et al. A randomized controlled trial of an alternative care provider clinic for severe sleep-disordered breathing. *Ann Am Thorac Soc.* 2019;16(12):1558-1566.
25. Bruyneel M. Telemedicine in the diagnosis and treatment of sleep apnoea. *Eur Respir Rev.* 2019; 28(151):180093.
26. Verbraecken J. Telemedicine applications in sleep disordered breathing: thinking out of the box. *Sleep Med Clin.* 2016;11(4):445-459.
27. Goldstein CA, Berry RB, Kent DT, et al. Artificial intelligence in sleep medicine: background and implications for clinicians. *J Clin Sleep Med.* 2020;16(4):609-618.
28. Malhotra A, Ayappa I, Ayas N, et al. Metrics of sleep apnea severity: beyond the AHI. *Sleep.* 2021; 44(7):zsab030.
29. Perez-Pozuelo I, Zhai B, Palotti J, et al. The future of sleep health: a data-driven revolution in sleep science and medicine. *NPJ Digit Med.* 2020;3:42.
30. Parthasarathy S, Guerra S, Quan S, et al. Does a peer support program improve satisfaction with treatment among patients with obstructive sleep apnea? Patient-Centered Outcomes Research Institute (PCORI). Available at: https://www.pcori.org/research-results/2013/does-peer-support-program-improve-satisfaction-treatment-among-patients-obstructive-sleep-apnea. Accessed March 1, 2024.
31. Riley S, Riley C. The role of patient navigation in improving the value of oncology care. *J Clin Pathways.* 2016;2(1):41-47.
32. Gieselmann A, Pietrowsky R. The effects of brief chat-based and face-to-face psychotherapy for insomnia: a randomized waiting list controlled trial. *Sleep Med.* 2019;61:63-72.
33. Seyffert M, Lagisetty P, Landgraf J, et al. Internet-delivered cognitive behavioral therapy to treat insomnia: a systematic review and meta-analysis. *PLoS One.* 2016;11(2):e0149139.
34. Hsieh C, Rezayat T, Zeidler MR. Telemedicine and the management of insomnia. *Sleep Med Clin.* 2020;15(3):383-390.
35. Bruyneel M. Technical developments and clinical use of telemedicine in sleep medicine. *J Clin Med.* 2016;5(12):116.
36. Hwang D, Chang JW, Benjafield AV, et al. Effect of telemedicine education and telemonitoring on continuous positive airway pressure adherence. The Tele-OSA Randomized Trial. *Am J Respir Crit Care Med.* 2018;197(1):117-126.
37. Kotzian ST, Schwarzinger A, Haider S, et al. Home polygraphic recording with telemedicine monitoring for diagnosis and treatment of sleep apnoea in stroke (HOPES Study): study protocol for a single-blind, randomised controlled trial. *BMJ Open.* 2018;8(1):e018847.
38. Nilius G, Schroeder M, Domanski U, et al. Telemedicine improves continuous positive airway pressure adherence in stroke patients with obstructive sleep apnea in a randomized trial. *Respiration.* 2019;98(5):410-420.
39. Murase K, Tanizawa K, Minami T, et al. A randomized controlled trial of telemedicine for long-term sleep apnea continuous positive airway pressure management. *Ann Am Thorac Soc.* 2020;17(3):329-337.
40. Aardoom JJ, Loheide-Niesmann L, Ossebaard HC, Riper H. Effectiveness of eHealth interventions in improving treatment adherence for adults with obstructive sleep apnea: meta-analytic review. *J Med Internet Res.* 2020;22(2):e16972.
41. Cervenka T, Iber C. EHR integration of PAP devices in sleep medicine implementation in the clinical setting. *Sleep Med Clin.* 2020;15(3):377-382.
42. Elson EC, Oermann C, Duehlmeyer S, Bledsoe S. Use of telemedicine to provide clinical pharmacy services during the SARS-CoV-2 pandemic. *Am J Health Syst Pharm.* 2020;77(13):1005-1006.
43. Correard F, Montaleytang M, Costa M, et al. Impact of medication review via tele-expertise on unplanned hospitalizations at 3 months of nursing homes patients (TEM-EHPAD): study protocol for a randomized controlled trial. *BMC Geriatr.* 2020;20(1):147.
44. Patient-Centered Outcomes Research Institute. Training Peer Buddies to Support Patients with Sleep Apnea. Available at: https://www.pcori.org/research-results/2019/training-peer-buddies-support-patients-sleep-apnea. Accessed March 1, 2024.

45. Zughni LA, Gillespie AI, Hatcher JL, et al. Telemedicine and the interdisciplinary clinic model: during the COVID-19 pandemic and beyond. *Otolaryngol Head Neck Surg*. 2020;163(4):673-675.
46. Funderskov KF, Boe Danbjorg D, Jess M, et al. Telemedicine in specialised palliative care: healthcare professionals' and their perspectives on video consultations—A qualitative study. *J Clin Nurs*. 2019;28 (21-22):3966-3976.
47. Provost K, Hilbert J. Home-based mechanical ventilation and neuromuscular disease: new horizons in home ventilation. *Chest Physician*: MDedge; 2021:23.

CHAPTER 6

Patient Education and Engagement for Telemedicine

Arveity R. Setty ■ Jennifer Dorsch ■ Charles J. Bae

Approximately 76% of U.S. hospitals engage in some form of telemedicine (TM), predominantly for radiology, psychiatry, or cardiology services.[1,2] However, TM composed a small percentage of out-patient practice before the coronavirus disease 2019 (COVID-19) public health emergency according to a 2018 study that reported only about 15.4% of physicians working in practices that used TM.[1] According to U.S. Centers for Disease Control and Prevention (CDC) reports, there was a 154% increase in telehealth visits during the last week in March 2020 compared with the same week in March 2019.[3] Sleep medicine was one of the early adopters, with 76% of visits from March 15 to May 8, 2020 with the primary complaint of "sleep disorder" occurring virtually.[4] Furthermore, the transition from in-person visits to virtual visits was made easier by the underlying infrastructure that was in place prior to the pandemic. A position paper published in 2015 by the American Association of Sleep Medicine (AASM) supported the use of TM for sleep complaints as long as minimum technological, diagnostic, safety, and privacy standards were met.[5] This consensus statement was made regarding the provision of specialty sleep medicine care to areas where it was otherwise unavailable, but it provided some guidance for large-scale implementation of TM, which was used during the COVID-19 public health crisis. Further strengthening rapid implementation of virtual visits during the pandemic, the AASM *SleepTM* virtual visit platform was rolled out in 2016 through the Veterans Administration with overwhelming success.[6] A recent update to the 2015 AASM position statement, published in the February 2021 edition of the *Journal of Clinical Sleep Medicine*, expands and updates the topics covered in the initial paper.[7]

After experiencing TM, both patients and providers are hesitant to give up this novel and convenient form of health care. In fact, 74% of patients who have used TM visits report high satisfaction.[8] Furthermore, as health equity becomes a goal of health care delivery, the TM infrastructure can be used to provide access to care to increasing numbers of patients, including those living in underserved communities. As of 2017, approximately 20% of the U.S. population resided in rural areas, and only 9% of physicians served these areas, causing a relative paucity of specialist care.[9] As a result, many practices are developing a hybrid model in which patients can be seen in person or virtually. Moving forward, it will be very important to determine what types of patients as well as what types of health problems are best treated in person versus virtually.

As virtual visits become more ubiquitous in sleep medicine practice, time and resources must be dedicated to preparing patients and providers for this mode of interaction to facilitate the delivery of optimal health care. Currently, patients are used to the traditional model of care, which is delivered in person and requires travel to an office or hospital setting. In this model, patients are instructed about different requirements and expectations before the visit, starting with a confirmation call or text message, a request to arrive 15 to 30 minutes before the scheduled visit to take care of administrative issues, and possibly a request for the patient to fill out pre-visit questionnaires. The goal of a virtual visit is to approximate an in-person visit as closely as possible, which means the tasks that were historically completed while the patient was physically in the office must be done in the virtual space. A study by Holtz showed that overall patients are satisfied with TM, but new users had slightly lower satisfaction compared with patients who were familiar with the virtual platform.[10] Therefore, especially for patients new to TM, expectations and instructions must be managed to provide a high-quality patient experience and health care.

We will discuss the infrastructure and employee education required for successful implementation of TM programs, how to educate and prepare patients for TM visits, methods for a smooth TM visit, and how to handle follow-up and intervisit communication and testing.

Types of Telemedicine Visits

First and foremost, the practice must evaluate their patient population, staff ability, technological support, and physician buy-in while they weigh the benefits and risks of offering TM. If the practice decides to proceed, the first decision that should be made is what type of virtual visit(s) will be offered as this will determine the infrastructure required for the interactions. Types of TM visits include synchronous live audio and audiovisual visits as well as asynchronous appointments.

AUDIO APPOINTMENTS

The least complicated visit would be an audio-only visit via telephone. This mode is the least cumbersome and requires only a telephone connection and a patient who is able to use a phone. This type of interaction foregoes most of the physical examination, only allowing for limited language and mental status assessments. This may negatively influence decision-making as well as make it more challenging to establish a patient-provider relationship. Another potential drawback is that this is the least reimbursed type of TM visit in the U.S. health system.

AUDIOVISUAL APPOINTMENTS

The second broad category of TM visit is the synchronous audiovisual appointment, which is based on a two-way connection between the patient and provider through the use of a camera and microphone. By incorporating the visual aspect, this type of visit allows for a limited physical examination and, in the United States, better reimbursement by insurance providers. This type of appointment requires more institutional support and patient buy-in to make it fruitful when compared with audio-only appointments.

Synchronous live interactions using a center-to-home (C2H) model means that there is a real-time audiovisual connection between the provider and patient and that the patient is located outside of a health care facility during the visit. The provider can be located at the health care facility or another location. With this model, patients are ultimately the ones who are responsible for connecting to the virtual visit platform using their own audiovisual-capable communication device such as a laptop, tablet, or smart phone. Benefits of the C2H model include ease of access for the patient if able to connect to the platform and lower implementation costs. The drawbacks include the risk of a privacy breach, difficulty with utilizing technology, and connectivity issues.[11]

Using the center-to-center (C2C) model, the patient physically comes to a collaborating provider's office or approved space while the consulting provider is located at another site. This type of model can be less convenient to patients and more resource intensive in that it requires a remote site agreement. On the plus side, it potentially provides improved privacy along with a higher-quality connection and technology.[11] The C2C model can allow more access to care for patients who do not have the proper equipment or connectivity, are technologically challenged, or live in a specialty provider–limited area.[12] When the patient arrives at the designated facility, a nurse or medical assistant will greet the patient and take their vital signs. There often is also a brief review of medications and the problem to be addressed at the visit, or chief complaint is elicited. Additional objective information such as weight and neck circumference can be obtained in this type of visit. Another benefit to the C2C model is that staff members who are trained on the technology and audiovisual platform can troubleshoot technical difficulties more easily.

ASYNCHRONOUS APPOINTMENTS

Asynchronous appointments refer to those in which information is uploaded to a virtual platform by a patient or health care provider to be reviewed by specialists and consultants at a future time for the purpose of diagnosis and management of a medical condition. Data transmitted to providers can take the form of images, videos, patient history, questions, or sleep-specific entities such as positive airway pressure compliance reports, sleep studies done at outside facilities, or sleep diaries. This type of interaction is also referred to as the *store-and-forward* method of interaction. If primary care providers are uploading the necessary information, then patients do not have much responsibility. However, if patients are partaking in the asynchronous visit, then they are responsible for uploading the necessary documents or images to the portal, which requires some degree of technological know-how, an Internet connection, potentially a cell phone with a camera for capturing images, and/or a scanner or scanner app for uploading paper documents.

Technology Infrastructure

Audio-only visits can be accomplished using the same resources as utilized during a routine phone call. One caveat is that if providers are calling from their personal phones, oftentimes number-masking technology is used so their personal phone number is not displayed to patients. This can be accomplished through telehealth apps, which will display the practice phone number as the originating number, or "*69," which causes the phone number to be blocked or "unknown." If the phone number used to make the call is blocked, then the patient should be notified that this is the case, as many individuals do not answer calls from blocked or "unknown" numbers.

When pursuing audiovisual visits, the chosen virtual platform must be easy to use, require limited knowledge of technology to implement, be Health Insurance Portability and Accountability Act (HIPAA)-compliant, and be reliable. There are many HIPAA-compliant virtual visit platforms available. In order to ensure adequate connectivity and save time during the patient encounter, office staff should prepare patients for their visit beforehand. During the pre-visit phone call, the individual responsible for check-in can inquire as to whether the patient has the technology to do a C2H visit, and if not, the provider should be alerted to that fact. Alternatives to C2H visits include in-person visits or converting to a telephone encounter. If the patient has the technology to do a C2H visit (i.e., a computer or smart phone with microphone and camera capabilities), then the check-in staff member should walk the patient through how to connect to the virtual visit. During this time, it is helpful for the staff to have a premade tip sheet detailing the step-by-step connection process along with common connectivity issues and troubleshooting tips to help patients connect to their virtual appointment.

Preparation for a Telemedicine Encounter

IDENTIFYING APPROPRIATE PATIENTS

It is important to identify patients who are appropriate for TM visits, and this can be done using two separate pathways. First, providers and staff must identify patients who are appropriate for TM encounters, and secondly patients can self-select for virtual visits after receiving education regarding the availability of TM appointments. Follow-up appointments for common sleep complaints such as insomnia, narcolepsy, idiopathic hypersomnolence, well-controlled obstructive

TABLE 6.1 ■ Criteria to Identify an Appropriate Patient for Telemedicine Visits

- Patient has the equipment (e.g., computer, smart phone, tablet) needed to access the TM platform.
- Patient has reliable access via Wi-Fi or cell service.
- Patient has knowledge of technology and ability to connect to the virtual platform. If not, patient has a family member or friend who is available to assist the patient if needed.
- Patient speaks English. If not, there is a translation service available for patients who speak another language or use sign language.
- Patient has a safe and private place in which to participate in the TM visit.
- Patient has a sleep disorder that does not require an in-person physical examination.

TM, Telemedicine.

sleep apnea, or CPAP compliance checks lend themselves well to TM visits because a physical examination is less important to the diagnosis and management of these conditions. New patient visits and sleep conditions that would benefit from in-person evaluation, such as poorly controlled sleep apnea due to mask leak or REM and behavior disorder with concern for development of an alpha-synucleinopathy, would not be good candidates for TM visits. Furthermore, patients with limited or unreliable Internet or phone access or patients who are unable to use the TM platform would be best served by in-person visits. To identify appropriate patients for TM visits, a check-list of criteria should be provided to schedulers, front desk staff, and providers (Table 6.1).

ADVERTISEMENT

When advertising for TM visits, effort should be made to directly educate patients, but also to notify local referral sources such as bariatric clinics, cardiology offices, or primary care physician offices of the availability of TM visits. Utilization of the practice website to advertise availability of TM visits can reach both referral sources and patients themselves, but it should be made clear that TM visits are only offered to specific patients and that patients or providers should call to inquire if they meet the criteria for TM appointments. If this strategy is utilized, then schedulers must be well trained on the availability for virtual visits, times these visits are offered, and criteria that must be met to allow for a virtual visit. The best way to standardize information that patients receive is to develop a script for the schedulers to use. Additionally, there should be a reference with answers to commonly asked questions related to TM visits provided to schedulers and front desk staff. Fliers can be distributed to patients who come for in-person appointments, and provid-ers can discuss the option for TM follow-up appointments at the close of new patient visits for appropriate patients. New patient introductory material can be sent electronically or via postal service and could include fliers advertising TM appointments and encouraging patients to ask their provider if a follow-up TM appointment is appropriate.

Patient Education Regarding Telemedicine Visits

When a TM visit is scheduled, the patient should receive information about the process of engag-ing in a TM visit as well as the practice's expectations for the visit. It should be made clear that TM visits are meant to mirror in-person appointments and that patients are expected to appear on camera in appropriate clothing, be in a location that is safe and conducive to a medical appoint-ment (e.g., a place that is private, not while the patient is driving), and be in a suitable state of mind to engage in a virtual visit. The patient should also be educated on the type of visit (audio-only visit, synchronous audiovisual visit using C2H or C2C, or asynchronous audiovisual visit) and how to engage in the visit. For audio-only visits, generally patients should be notified that a medical assistant or staff member will be contacting them prior to the appointment for check-in, at which point they will be asked questions about insurance, reason for the visit, and center-specific questions such as medication reconciliation or the Epworth Sleepiness Scale. After check-in, patients should be instructed that they will receive a phone call from the provider to discuss their medical condition and its diagnosis or treatment. For synchronous audiovisual visit using C2H model, patients should be notified about how they will receive the link to the virtual meeting (i.e., via email or text message) and if there are any applications that must be downloaded prior to the appointment to support those platforms. At this point, it may be beneficial to explain that recent studies have shown that TM visits have similar efficacy when compared with in-person visits in a variety of health care situations such as mental health care and dermatology appointments.[13] Additionally, studies evaluating sleep-specific medical conditions such as obstructive sleep apnea[14-16] and insomnia[17] have demonstrated successful treatment of these conditions using telehealth, which may encourage TM visits or ease any apprehensions regarding this model of visit.

Check-In

As mentioned earlier, the time leading to the appointment should mimic in-person appointments as closely as possible. For many practices, once patients arrive at clinic, they are roomed, medications are verified, CPAP downloads are obtained, and the Epworth Sleepiness Scale is administered. These things are still done in the virtual space during the check-in process. Instead of downloading CPAP compliance reports from a physical USB chip, support staff can query cloud-based databases for compliance reports and upload them to the patient's chart during this time if not done already. During the check-in process, support staff (clerical staff, medical assistant, or nurse) can help with troubleshooting connection problems if needed and verify patient location and safety for the visit. Check-in can happen with a phone call or in the virtual room before the provider portion of the visit.

The Provider Encounter

The workflow for the virtual provider encounter is very similar to in-person visits; however, there are some advantages to virtual visits. One study evaluating telehealth visits versus standard of care for pre-surgical assessments found that telehealth visits were on average 20 minutes shorter than in-person visits.[18] When looking at patient-per-hour rate, a study of emergency departments utilizing telehealth to screen patients did not find a statistical difference between telehealth and in-person visits, but fewer patients left without being seen in the in-person screening arm compared with the telehealth arm.[19] This is important to keep in mind because, much like in-person visits, providers can run behind schedule during TM visits. Methods such as messaging patients to notify them when providers are running behind schedule and pre-appointment counseling regarding potential delays could reduce patient impatience and angst.

Wrap-Up

After the encounter is complete, the provider must signal to the office staff that the patient is ready to be "checked out." This can be accomplished using email, features of the virtual visit platform, or even on the electronic medical record (EMR) if it is supported. After the office staff receives notice that the appointment has concluded and that appropriate orders for testing, referrals, and return visits have been placed, then the patient can be contacted to make follow-up appointments if needed.

Intervisit Communication

Patients who engage in TM visits typically demonstrate the technological know-how necessary for portal-based communication. Oftentimes, secure messaging is the easiest and most time-efficient method for patients and staff to ask questions, provide follow-up information, or inform others about difficulties or lapses in treatment. Patients should be told of the standard response times and informed of approximately what time and frequency messages are checked and addressed.

Conclusion

TM appointments have become commonplace following the COVID-19 pandemic. Based on ease of use, patient and provider satisfaction, and availability of suitable virtual platforms, it is likely that this mode of patient care delivery will play a central role in the evolution and expansion of sleep medicine. To ensure optimal care, patients and providers must be educated on how to best utilize this modality of health care delivery. Working toward this goal, training programs are starting to include TM education as part of their curricula.[20,21] Office staff and providers convey crucial information regarding TM to patients and play a key role in setting expectations.

References

1. Kane CK, Gillis K. The use of telemedicine by physicians: still the exception rather than the rule. *Health Aff (Millwood)*. 2018;37(12):1923-1930.
2. Hyder MA, Razzak J. Telemedicine in the United States: an introduction for students and residents. *J Med Internet Res*. 2020;22(11):e20839.
3. Koonin LM. Trends in the use of telehealth during the emergence of the COVID-19 pandemic — United States, January–March 2020. *MMWR Morb Mortal Wkly Rep*. 2020;69(43):1595-1599.
4. Fox B, Sizemore JO. *As Office Visits Fall, Telehealth Takes Hold*. Epic Health Research Network; 2021. Available at: https://ehrn.org/articles/as-office-visits-fall-telehealth-takes-hold/. Accessed March 1, 2024.
5. Singh J, Badr MS, Diebert W, et al. American Academy of Sleep Medicine (AASM) position paper for the use of telemedicine for the diagnosis and treatment of sleep disorders. *J Clin Sleep Med*. 2015; 11(10):1187-1198.
6. Watson NF. Expanding patient access to quality sleep health care through telemedicine. *J Clin Sleep Med*. 2016;12(2):155-156.
7. Shamim-Uzzaman QA, Bae CJ, Ehsan Z, et al. The use of telemedicine for the diagnosis and treatment of sleep disorders: an American Academy of Sleep Medicine update. *J Clin Sleep Med*. 2021;17(5): 1103-1107.
8. Meet-The-Rising-Bar-For-Virtual-Patient-Experience. Available at: https://www.advisory.com/Topics/Patient-Experience-and-Satisfaction/2020/10/Meet-The-Rising-Bar-For-Virtual-Patient-Experience. Accessed March 1, 2024.
9. Gudbranson E, Glickman A, Emanuel EJ. Reassessing the data on whether a physician shortage exists. *JAMA*. 2017;317(19):1945.
10. Holtz BE. Patients perceptions of telemedicine visits before and after the Coronavirus Disease 2019 pandemic. *Telemed J E Health*. 2020;27(1):107-112.
11. Khosla S. Implementation of synchronous telemedicine into clinical practice. *Sleep Med Clin*. 2020; 15(3):347-358.
12. Watson NF, Rosen IM, Chervin RD. The past is prologue: the future of sleep medicine. *J Clin Sleep Med*. 2017;13(1):127-135.
13. Shigekawa E, Fix M, Corbett G, et al. The current state of telehealth evidence: a rapid review. *Health Aff (Millwood)*. 2018;37(12):1975-1982.
14. Schutte-Rodin S. Telehealth, telemedicine, and obstructive sleep apnea. *Sleep Med Clin*. 2020;15(3):359-375.

15. Bruyneel M. Telemedicine in the diagnosis and treatment of sleep apnoea. *Eur Respir Rev.* 2019; 28(151):180093.
16. Lugo VM, Garmendia O, Suarez-Girón M, et al. Comprehensive management of obstructive sleep apnea by telemedicine: clinical improvement and cost-effectiveness of a virtual sleep unit. a randomized controlled trial. *PLoS One.* 2019;14(10):e0224069.
17. Gieselmann A, Pietrowsky R. The effects of brief chat-based and face-to-face psychotherapy for insomnia: a randomized waiting list controlled trial. *Sleep Med.* 2019;61:63-72.
18. Mullen-Fortino M, Rising KL, Duckworth J, et al. Presurgical assessment using telemedicine technology: impact on efficiency, effectiveness, and patient experience of care. *Telemed J E Health.* 2019;25(2):137-142.
19. Rademacher NJ, Cole G, Psoter KJ, et al. Use of telemedicine to screen patients in the emergency department: matched cohort study evaluating efficiency and patient safety of telemedicine. *JMIR Med Inform.* 2019;7(2):e11233.
20. Walker C, Echternacht H, Brophy PD. Model for medical student introductory telemedicine education. *Telemed J E Health.* 2019;25(8):717-723.
21. Ainslie M, Bragdon C. Telemedicine simulation in online family nurse practitioner education: clinical competency and technology integration. *J Am Assoc Nurse Pract.* 2018;30(8):430-434.

CHAPTER 7

Fellowship and Training

Ian D. Weir ▓ Santosh Vaghela ▓ Hira Bakhtiar

Telehealth and Medical Education

Virtual Clinical Care and Didactic Delivery in a Virtual Clinical Learning Environment

Although the field of sleep medicine seems well positioned for telemedicine, sleep fellowship programs have not universally adopted telemedicine care delivery by trainees. For example, a survey study conducted prior to the coronavirus disease 2019 (COVID-19) pandemic by Fields et al.[1] demonstrated that 33.3% of the sleep fellowship program directors (PDs) offer telemedicine experience to their trainees, although none use a standard telemedicine curriculum. Among the 66.7% PDs not offering a telemedicine experience, 38.5% plan to do so, and 53.9% agree that it would benefit fellows. New payer policies have made telemedicine services more accessible for patients, and the Accreditation Council for Graduate Medical Education (ACGME) now permits telemedicine to be incorporated into clinical training programs.[2,3] These recent changes help sleep medicine fellowships facilitate the opportunity to provide trainees with skills needed during their professional careers. In this chapter, we will dive into specific aspects of sleep medicine training in telehealth—how to conduct a visit with a trainee, curriculum and training, evaluation and feedback, and using virtual and distance learning methods.

Core Requirements of Telehealth Training in Sleep Fellowship

It is prudent to have trainees engage in a formal training curriculum for telemedicine visits prior to seeing patients on their respective platforms. Development of "webside manner" has become paramount in the 21st century as telemedicine continues to flourish (see Chapter 9). Medical schools have embraced the need to deliver care remotely, and several have incorporated teaching telemedicine into their basic science and clinical training.[4] Training in telehealth during sleep fellowship calls for a structured and defined format as well as a platform to provide quality medical care, maintain efficiency, and incorporate meaningful education for learners. There is also a need for assessment of perceived importance or relevance of telehealth, knowledge of telehealth services, and comfort in providing telehealth services and perceived barriers to using telehealth in the future. Integration of telemedicine services requires implementation of a formal telemedicine training, which involves undergoing orientation to the platform and consultation process, shadowing attending physicians using telemedicine, and participating in tele-sleep case conferences. Such curricula may serve as models for integrating telemedicine education into other residency and training programs. Unfortunately, no evidence-based data exist to guide programs on the optimal way to teach or incorporate trainees into telehealth. To this effect, information in this chapter serves as a descriptive guide and reference to which programs may build their own sleep medicine telehealth curriculum and clinical experience.

TABLE 7.1 ■ Implementation of Telemedicine Curriculum for Sleep Medicine

Curriculum	Learning Telecommunicative Technology	Digital Diagnostics Learning	Webside Manners
• Modules • Lectures • Simulation training • Case-based E-learning	• Electronic platform used at the training institution	• Diagnostics: PSG reading virtually • Getting comfortable to navigate the platform	• Positioning the video camera • Nonverbal cues • Effective engagement of patients • Oversight

PSG, Polysomnography.

Table 7.1 provides an example of a format to effectively implement telemedicine curriculum that utilizes learning modules for successful telemedicine technology education; it is always helpful to give lectures about the history of telemedicine, how it works, and learning aspects on how to utilize telemedicine, which are more relevant for trainees preparing to enter the physician workforce. Integrating telemedicine into graduate medical education (GME) curricula provides an important mechanism for improving trainee education on value-based care and increasing access to specialty care. It is also equally important to learn the technology around telemedicine. A digital learning environment can also be used to navigate polysomnography readings as well as other aspects of sleep medicine.

These courses can include lectures, shadowing physicians working in telehealth clinics, simulated video encounters with standardized patients, students interviewing patients over a video monitor, and learning how to take a medical history remotely. These sessions also include feedback from faculty that can help fine-tune the encounters for trainees. On-demand sessions may be pre-recorded and placed in the institution's cloud server for immediate access to refresh on topics or issues that may arise as well. The American Academy of Sleep Medicine clinical resources web page provides the fellow with basic telehealth knowledge and is a helpful reference for sleep fellows starting their fellowships.[5]

Conducting a Telehealth Clinical Visit With a Trainee

The general framework for a teaching telehealth visit that includes a teaching faculty clinician and trainee (medical student, resident, or fellow) is similar to that for an in-person visit, but with a few important caveats. Many of these nuanced differences are addressed in this section. Although the authors do not endorse a specific platform for telehealth encounters, we will reference a commonly used platform only as an example of how the encounter may be completed. Specific issues to be addressed include trainee education, setting up patient visits, conducting a patient visit, staffing patients with the sleep faculty, documentation and billing of telehealth visits, and standardized training of early learners in telehealth encounters.

Setting up the Patient Visit

The telehealth visit requires a significant amount of preparation prior to the visit and on the day of the visit. This includes collection of data from the patient that will be useful for the day of the visit such as office forms, standardized questionnaires (such as Epworth Sleepiness Scale score), downloads from continuous positive airway pressure (CPAP) machines, and placement of all of these items into the electronic health record (EHR) to ensure that they are available to the clinical team on the day of the visit.

Reviewing Studies Beforehand

Similar to in-person visits, it is recommended that the trainee "pre-round" on the patient's chart to ensure that all necessary studies and documentation are available for the visit to be conducted smoothly. This includes but is not limited to ensuring that intake paperwork is available, standardized questionnaires are filled out, CPAP machine data are uploaded, and prior notes to address issues that may arise during the visit are reviewed. This will help streamline the visit and allow for an improved patient experience and productive virtual visit.

Day of the Visit

The teaching faculty must be available during the clinic hours scheduled and able to adequately participate in the telehealth visit. This includes verifying that the teaching faculty computer and/or mobile device is working, connected to the Internet, and able to log in to the telehealth platform as well as access the EHR. Additionally, a communications "back channel" is available for the trainee to access the faculty while not in front of the patient for addressing any clinical- or training-related concerns. This could include but is not limited to Health Insurance Portability and Accountability Act (HIPAA)-compliant texting, secure messaging via the EHR, phone calls, or other alternative means set in advance of the patient encounter.

A list of patients and visit times is available for the staff. At the designated time, the trainee logs in to the platform for the telehealth visit and verifies the patient's location, including city and state. The trainees obtain consent for the telehealth visit and confirm if anyone else is present with the patient for the visit or needs to be present for the visit to continue. The trainee also explains that the visit will be done as part of a teaching program, and an attending physician will be available for the key portions of the telehealth visit. Based on the individual faculty preference as well as clinic or hospital policies, the attending physician may be present for the entirety of the visit.

Seeing Patients

The visit is conducted in a standard patient assessment format that is similar to an in-person visit. The major differences may include allowing for technical issues/slowdowns with the telemedicine platform, troubleshooting issues with the video and/or audio, changing the cadence of speech for the platform chosen, and of course, conducting a virtual physical examination.

Reviewing Studies With the Patient

Some platforms, including the one that we use, allow for a "screen-sharing" function. This can be useful for the physician to review studies with the patient, similar to an in-person visit. We advocate for the trainee to have the patient's relevant studies up in the background of their computer and, at the appropriate time, to utilize the screen-sharing function on their platform to review the test results with the patient. The attending is available during this time to address any issues that may arise from the patient and to later provide feedback to the trainee in their counseling of the patient on their results.

Precepting With Faculty With the Patient on Hold

Once the interview is completed, the patient is notified that the trainee and the faculty clinician will confer about the patient's clinical condition. The audio and video from the microphone and camera are muted during this time, and the trainee and faculty can discuss the findings either in person, by phone, or utilizing a "waiting room" feature of the telehealth platform. As is done in most in-person examinations, the "staffing" of the patient is one of the most crucial aspects to the training experience and is no different in the telemedicine platform. In addition to providing feedback and guidance regarding clinical medicine, the attending will discuss the trainee's appearance on the telehealth audio and visual and provide additional feedback as needed. This will help trainees fine-tune their future visits to allow for more streamlined visits.

Completing the Visit

Once the staffing of the patient is complete, both the trainee and faculty return to the camera, turn the audio and visual back on, and discuss the plan with the patient. Adequate time is given to allow for any questions to be answered, as for any in-person visit. It should be decided beforehand who will lead this portion of the visit as most telemedicine platforms only allow one speaker at a time. To complete the interview, the patient can be removed to either a virtual waiting room, or the visit can simply end. As with any in-person visit, documentation will need to be completed after the visit as well as orders and a subsequent follow-up plan.

Special Considerations for Telehealth Clinical Visits Conducted With a Trainee

There is no universally accepted way to conduct telehealth clinical visits with sleep trainees. Each individual fellowship program will need to take into account its own telehealth platform capabilities and limitations, faculty experience and preference, and logistical concerns to design a workflow that meets their needs. Telehealth allows for flexibility, and many options exist. In one approach, the sleep faculty and trainee are each physically present in different rooms within the out-patient clinic; in another, all participants are in different physical locations. The sleep faculty could be present for the entire visit (with a visit break for the fellow and attending to confer), providing further opportunity for the attending to observe the fellow's history-building and communication skills. This kind of direct observation is a potential benefit of the telemedicine environment, as the faculty's presence is not as physically intrusive as it might be during in-person visits. In general, incorporating a sleep trainee into clinical visits is feasible and has advantages and disadvantages over face-to-face visits. A structured format may help standardize telehealth visits across the clinical care within the sleep fellowship training program.

Billing Telehealth Visits With a Trainee

Outpatient Evaluation and Management (E/M) coding and documentation reforms took effect on January 1, 2021, and now allow physicians and other qualified health professionals (QHPs) to code office visits based solely on total time.[6] In our experience, this is the most common way to support E/M coding for out-patient telehealth. Although a full discussion of billing is beyond the scope of this chapter, there are a few important considerations when a trainee is involved with the clinical visit.[7] First, the faculty physician and other QHPs, not the trainee, sign and submit the bill. Second, time spent teaching the trainee does not count toward the total encounter time. Third, time spent between the trainee and patient without the faculty present (virtual or in person) does not count toward the total time. And lastly, the sleep faculty must attest and document total encounter time. Billing rules and their interpretation by institutions change frequently, and it is advised to consult with your coding and compliance department for further guidance (Figure 7.1).

Trainee Feedback and Evaluation

Use of a telehealth format allows for direct observation of the trainee-patient encounter by faculty and is ideally suited for evaluating trainees and providing effective feedback. Opportunities to

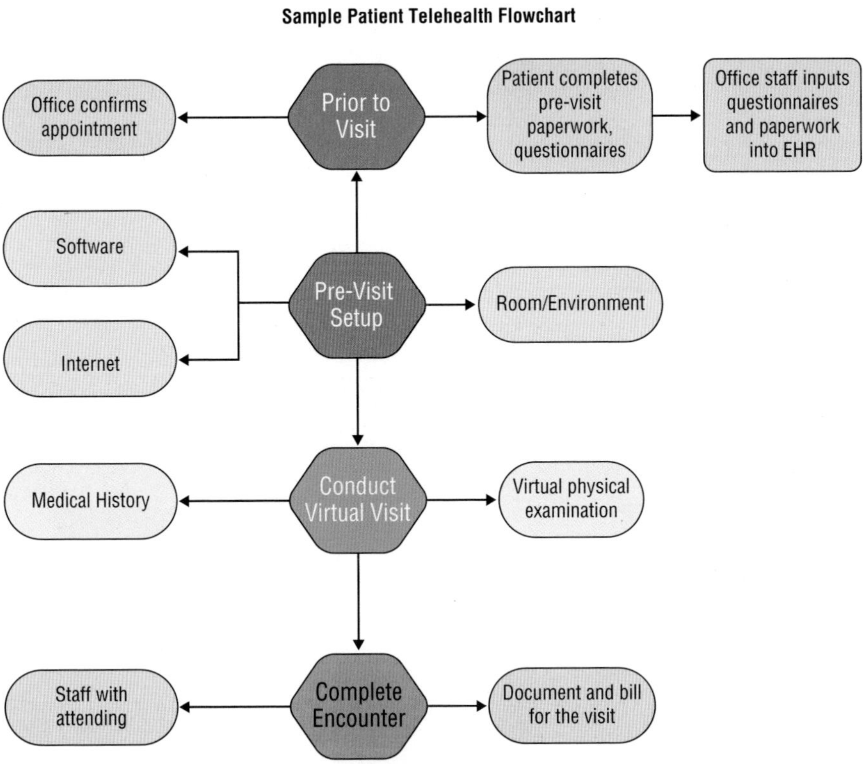

Sample Patient Telehealth Flowchart

Figure 7.1 A sample telemedicine flowchart for organizations to use in a teaching environment. *EHR,* Electronic health record.

assess history-gathering and communication skills via telehealth align well with fundamental components of competency-based medical education, including patient care, interpersonal and communication skills, and faculty feedback. Figure 7.2 highlights some of the trainee factors that are helpful for best telemedicine practices during training. Additionally, there are important and unique skills in conducting telehealth visits that could be assessed by a dedicated telehealth evaluation. Sleep fellowship programs may wish to create a trainee telehealth evaluation to incorporate into their evaluation methods. One such telehealth evaluation is referenced in Table 7.2 and available in the appendix. It may be used and edited to suit individual program needs. Providing effective feedback to the trainee is an important element of a sleep training program. Although providing feedback after a directly observed telehealth patient encounter should not be much different than in person, a structured format and expectations are helpful to facilitate the process. If the virtual platform, patient, and institution allow session recording, attending physicians can provide feedback via post hoc review of fellow-delivered care as an alternative to mini-clinical examination (Mini-CEX); fellows may gain new insights into their care delivery by viewing a video of themselves engaged in real-world virtual patient care. Additionally, patient experience and trainee performance survey data from patients can be collected and provide important information to help provide feedback. In summary, directly observed telehealth encounters allow an opportunity to build skills and enhance performance of the trainee through evaluation and feedback.

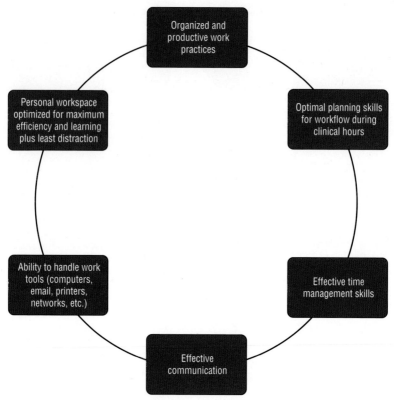

Figure 7.2   Trainee factors that are helpful for best telemedicine practices.

Virtual Learning

With the COVID-19 pandemic came a rapid shift toward virtual learning that was unprecedented in GME. In addition to clinical exposure and training, sleep fellowship programs must provide adequate didactics and scholarship. A broad range of didactic activities is a core component of fellowship training curricula. These include lectures, case conferences, grand rounds, simulations, case-based teaching, and journal clubs. Although traditionally occurring in person, virtual platforms allow programs to continue structured educational curricula while complying with physical distancing directives and have been met with varying levels of satisfaction due to inherent advantages and disadvantages. For an excellent review of this topic, we suggest the article by Shelgkar entitled "Optimizing Virtual and Distance Learning During an Emergency and Beyond."[8] Anecdotally, many physicians have observed and reported an increase in conference attendance as faculty members, emeritus staff, community physicians, public health experts, and others who are traditionally unable to attend have engaged with learners, bringing different perspectives and expertise that strengthen discussions. Virtual platforms have accelerated the adoption of alternative teaching methods, like team-based learning, that promote active learning. "Breakout room" features facilitate team-based learning by allowing learners to be pushed electronically to smaller groups and then back together to the same larger virtual room instantaneously. We have found that the time investment required to learn and master the basic and advanced features of virtual platforms

TABLE 7.2 ■ **Examples of a Telehealth Trainee Evaluation**

Sleep Medicine Fellow Telehealth—Expectations
Listed on this form are the specific expectations for telehealth training as specified in the Sleep
  Medicine Fellowship Curriculum. Fellows will be expected to add these skills, practices, attitudes,
  and knowledge in subsequent months as specified in the curriculum.
Please rate the fellow's performance of the items listed below.
1. Medical knowledge
  a. Is able to conduct a telehealth visit from start to finish
  b. Understands the limitations of telehealth for sleep patients
  c. Demonstrates knowledge of the regulatory requirements for telehealth
  d. Demonstrates comprehensive skills conducting a telehealth visit
  e. Documents in the EMR are the necessary verbiage for a telehealth visit
2. Patient care
  a. Provides comprehensive sleep evaluation and diagnosis along with treatment planning to adults
    and children with sleep complaints
  b. Is sensitive to patients' needs, cultural background, and individual preferences in their care
  c. Uses available resources to educate patients and their families and is proactive in teaching them
    about sleep
  d. Has developed a clinical alliance with patients
  e. Provides clear, concise education about clinical data to patients and families in follow-up visits
3. Practice-based learning
  a. Patient and procedure logs reflect comprehensive training among a diversity of patient types as
    well as required procedures
  b. Collaborates in development of optimal patient care with technical staff and colleagues
4. Interpersonal and communication skills
  a. Demonstrates sensitivity to cultural issues of patients and their families during clinical encounters
  b. Conveys clinical information promptly, with consistent attention to important details and clarity of
    thought
  c. Demonstrates respect and open-mindedness during discussions with center staff, patients, and
    colleagues in performing clinical care for patients
5. Professionalism
  a. Displays respect, total commitment to self-assessment, willingness to acknowledge errors, and ele-
    vation of need to others above self-interest in the fellow's relationships with patients, peers, and staff
  b. Work ethic displays integrity that engenders the respect of colleagues
6. System-based learning
  a. Demonstrates clear understanding of the organization of homecare companies and conveys this
    to patients when helpful
  b. Initiates appropriate referrals to the other subspecialties, or contact with referring physician when
    necessary to provide patient follow-up
  c. Utilizes available clinical services for patient care effectively, with a realistic understanding of their
    contributions

EMR, Electronic medical record.

pays substantial dividends by enabling active learning during teaching sessions. In fact, more meticulous preparation in advance of virtual didactic sessions may result in more effective, well-delivered, and well-received presentations.

Lectures, case-based presentations, and other didactic offerings can still thrive in a distance learning environment. Many institutions have subscription agreements with virtual conferencing platforms that programs can use to convene trainees, faculty, and other members of the sleep team. Case conferences should be held only on platforms compliant with the HIPAA of 1996.

Virtual didactic offerings can broaden the scope of training programs, which now have a cost-effective means for their trainees to engage with clinical and research educators across the

TABLE 7.3 ■ **Advantages and Disadvantages of Online Didactics**

Advantages	Disadvantages
Flexible learning	Requires self-motivation and discipline
Creative teaching techniques	Limited networking and social interaction
Individualized learning	Asynchronous learning does not allow for real-time faculty-fellow interaction
Accessibility	Limited nonverbal communications
Convenience	Perception that virtual education is not as effective as traditional didactic teaching
Equal participation	Traditional instructors may be challenged and uncomfortable with technology
Anonymity	
Cost savings	

country and the globe. Incorporation of continuing medical education credit into virtual conferences can also attract other participants and broaden the reach of a training program's educational conferences.

Virtual learning does have significant drawbacks (Table 7.3). It is particularly difficult for presenters to recognize nonverbal cues in an audience that is often muted and not seen, leading to the analogy of a "blindfolded speaker." For trainees at earlier stages of teaching and presentation abilities, this can be especially challenging. We encourage PDs to coach trainees through this process and provide feedback. Online formats also limit the culture building and comradery essential to the well-being and mental health of faculty and learners. Increased mindfulness around and incorporation of morale-building activities may help overcome this reality. In addition, inevitable frustration and avoidance of participation can ensue for individuals who are not technologically adept, and even those with more skills can have a steep learning curve to utilize the full capabilities of the various platforms. It is not unreasonable to adopt a hybrid approach of limited in-person attendance based on institutional policy, combined with real-time video streaming of the interactive educational activity. In-person simulation exercises can be implemented using a role-play activity between two faculty members, one playing a provider with questions (the caller) and the other the expert providing answers (the provider carrying the pager). Fellows then engage in a pair-share activity to discuss their approach to the caller's questions, followed by debrief and feedback. Links to conferences could be shared with other departments or training programs, thereby providing fellows with additional opportunities to teach faculty, peers, and more junior learners. Enhanced telehealth capabilities and pandemic conditions have created the opportunity for a virtual learning environment. With careful attention to the advantages and disadvantages, these methods can enhance trainee education and satisfaction within the framework of the sleep medicine training program.

Conclusion

In this chapter, we discussed strategies to conduct a telehealth visit with a trainee, important elements of a structured telehealth curriculum, methods for feedback and evaluation of trainee telehealth performance, and the role of virtual learning. To prepare fellowship trainees for a successful career in sleep medicine, fellowship programs will need to embrace telehealth and virtual learning. Future evidence-based strategies should be developed to optimize telehealth training to guide sleep fellowship programs.

References

1. Fields BG, Dholakia SA, Ioachimescu OC. Sleep telemedicine training in fellowship programs: a survey of program directors. *J Clin Sleep Med.* 2020;16(4):575-581.
2. Centers for Medicare and Medicaid Services. Medicare Telemedicine Health Care Provider Fact Sheet. 2020. Available at: https://www.cms.gov/newsroom/fact-sheets/medicare-telemedicine-health-care-provider-fact-sheet. Accessed March 1, 2024.
3. Accreditation Council for Graduate Medical Education ACGME Response to COVID-19: Clarification regarding Telemedicine and ACGME Surveys. Available at: https://www.acgme.org/newsroom/blog/2020/3/acgme-response-to-covid-19-clarification-regarding-telemedicine-and-acgme-surveys/. Accessed March 1, 2024.
4. Chart on Number of Medical Schools Including Telemedicine in Curricula Source: LCME Annual Medical School Questionnaire Part II, 2014-2015 through 2019-2020. Available at: https://www.aamc.org/data-reports/curriculum-reports/data/curriculum-change-medical-schools. Accessed March 1, 2024.
5. Academy American of Sleep Medicine Telemedicine: American Academy of Sleep Medicine clinical resources. Available at: https://aasm.org/clinical-resources/telemedicine/telemedicine-faq/. Accessed March 1, 2024.
6. Centers for Medicare and Medicaid Services. Evaluation and Management Services Guide. Available at: Available at: https://www.cms.gov/outreach-and-education/medicare-learning-network-mln/mlnproducts/mln-publications-items/cms1243514. Accessed March 1, 2024.
7. Centers for Medicare, Services Medicaid Guidelines for Teaching Physicians, Interns, and Residents. Available at: https://www.cms.gov/outreach-and-education/medicare-learning-network-mln/mlnproducts/mln-publications-items/cms1243499. Accessed March 1, 2024.
8. Shelgkar AV. Optimizing virtual and distance learning during an emergency and beyond. *J Clin Sleep Med.* 2020;16(11):1929-1932.

Nuts and Bolts

CHAPTER 8

Determining Patient-Provider Suitability and Informed Consent

William F. Martin

Telemedicine is not new in the diagnosis and treatment of sleep disorders.[1] The novel coronavirus (SARS-CoV-2) and the coronavirus disease 2019 (COVID-19) accelerated ongoing trends in advances and adoption of sleep telemedicine.[2] Furthermore, this accelerated trend is expected to continue.[2] This trend in sleep medicine is reflected in other specialties. As an example, Medicare fee-for-service primary care visits provided via telehealth increased from <1% before the COVID-19 pandemic to greater than 60%[3] and remains a stable care delivery model for many practices.

Diversity: Patients, Providers, Settings, and Technology

There is diversity in the types of patients, types of providers, the settings in which telemedicine is used, and the technology associated with the provision and utilization of telemedicine. A brief review is warranted prior to narrowing down on the focus of this chapter: patient-provider suitability and informed consent. To determine suitability involves a decision that is made based on standards and the specific practice context as well as consideration of the features, benefits, and limits of specific telemedicine technologies.

PATIENT DIVERSITY

Patient characteristics of importance include the following: demographics, socioeconomic status including health insurance coverage, health literacy, digital literacy, and access to telemedicine technology and associated infrastructure such as adequate bandwidth.[4] All of these factors also relate to equity in telemedicine. Patient preference is another factor with findings suggesting that patients are more willing to use telemedicine if they have an existing relationship with the provider.[5]

PROVIDER DIVERSITY

Provider characteristics of importance include the following: cost, reimbursement, legal liability, privacy, confidentiality, data security, efficiency, and workflow.[6] A useful conceptual framework to predict, explain, and influence provider adoption of telemedicine is the technology acceptance model (TAM).[7] Figure 8.1 depicts the basic TAM. As shown in Figure 8.1, the external variables include patient characteristics, the setting, and the specific technology, not to mention the organizational context.

On close examination, providers are likely to perceive telemedicine to be suitable as a tool they will use based on their perceptions in two domains: usefulness of telemedicine and ease of use. These two factors will shape the attitude of providers toward their behavioral intent to actually use telemedicine. Actual telemedicine use is partially dependent on the factors presented in this framework. This model has been critiqued for being overly simplistic.[8] There are more

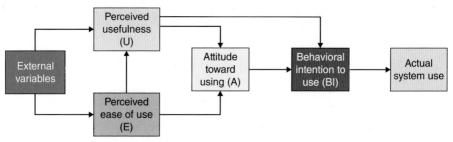

Figure 8.1 The basic technology acceptance model.

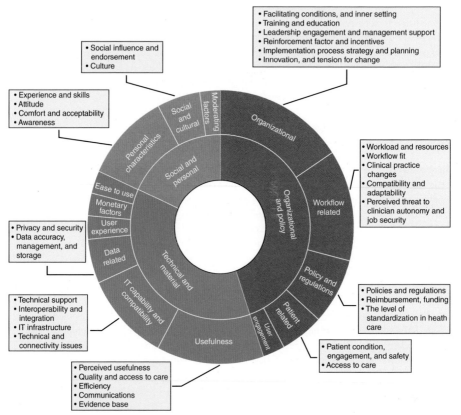

Figure 8.2 Consolidated framework of the factors affecting the clinician's adaptation of mobile health. *IT,* Information technology. *(From Jacob C, Sanchez-Vazquez A, Ivory C. Understanding clinicians' adoption of mobile health tools: a qualitative review of the most used frameworks. JMIR Mhealth Uhealth. 2020;8[7]:1-20, https://mhealth. jmir.org/2020/7/e18072).*

comprehensive models, such as the consolidated framework of the factors affecting clinicians' adaptation of mobile health.[9] Figure 8.2 shows the consolidated framework.

SETTING DIVERSITY

Setting characteristics are driven by patient factors, provider factors, telemedicine technology factors, legal/regulatory factors, reimbursement factors, and the type of telemedicine clinical encounter. Telemedicine clinical encounters include but are not limited to the following: E-consult; remote patient monitoring (RPT); patient-initiated messaging-synchronous or asynchronous; telephone visit; and video visit.[10] One limiting factor is that a thorough, comprehensive physical examination is not possible if the patient is at home, yet some aspects of the physical examination are possible.[11]

TELEMEDICINE TECHNOLOGY DIVERSITY

An optimal patient experience depends on high-quality communication between the patient and provider without interruptions in audio or voice.[12] Not all telemedicine technology is synchronous, such as consumer sleep technologies including apps and wearables. The American Academy of Sleep Medicine's Consumer Sleep Technology Position Statement[13] outlines advantages and disadvantages of this technology but recognizes that these technologies can be used to enhance patient engagement and the patient-provider interaction. Regarding wearables, evidence from a systematic review concludes that most wearables do not compare with polysomnography with regard to monitoring sleep reliably.[14]

Convergence: Patients, Providers, Settings, and Technology

All four of the aforementioned factors must be considered to inform these two decisions prior to being concerned about informed consent.

- Which type of telemedicine, if any, is suitable for the patient at this time?
- Which type of telemedicine, if any, is suitable for the provider for this patient at this time?

Both of these questions are framed to account for the relationship between the patient and provider and the particular context. Telemedicine may be determined to be suitable in one instance for a patient but not so in another instance with the very same patient. Telemedicine may also be a suitable option for a provider with a particular diagnosis, patient, or setting, but not with another diagnosis, patient, or setting.

CLINICAL VIGNETTE

A 54-year-old male patient employed at a call center with rotating shifts was recently diagnosed with obstructive sleep apnea (OSA). The patient is now trying to use continuous positive airway pressure (CPAP). He already had CPAP patient education but asked for the patient education materials to be mailed to his home. The patient informed the nurse that he did not know how to access the web-based OSA educational materials and that he does not check his email. The patient's use of CPAP is not routine. He reports that he needs help to use the CPAP regularly.

As the provider, you finished reading about a randomized trial using CPAP telemonitoring with automated patient feedback.[15] You ask the patient which type of feedback he prefers among the choices available: text messaging, email, phone call, or a combination. The patient chooses the phone call. As the provider, this was not your first option, but on further inquiry with the patient, you discover that the patient is low on digital literacy and lives in a community without high-quality bandwidth.

As depicted in this clinical vignette, the provider had to consider the patient characteristics that were facilitators or barriers to the patient adoption of three telemedicine technology tools. The challenge for the provider is that one of the barriers (i.e., digital literacy) can be addressed but begs the question as to whose role it is in the health care delivery system. The other barrier (i.e., low bandwidth in the community) is not likely to be considered part of the role and responsibility of the individual provider, but it is the role of the organization. These considerations are important because context matters, but they are beyond the scope of this chapter.

Informed Consent: Patient-Centered Care

Informed consent sits at the nexus of ethics and the law.[16] Patient-centered care "…is an approach to care and perceived as the right thing to do" (p. 101).[17] Philosophically, informed consent promotes personal autonomy or self-determination.[18] It is beyond the scope here to catalog the critiques of informed consent as merely disclosing information rather than seeking understanding by the patient in a way to promote shared decision-making. Shared decision-making is regarded as "the pinnacle of patient-centered care" (p. 780).[19] Informed consent is a foundational element of any patient encounter regardless of whether the visit is in person or mediated through technology.[20]

Informed Consent: Beyond the Standard Informed Consent

The decision by the patient to select in-person services and/or technology-mediated services should be based on information provided by the provider.[20] Hence, informed consent begins with a disclosure and discussion of the treatment options. Informed consent for in-person examinations, visits, consultations, and procedures typically focuses on the medical issue, treatment options, risks, and benefits. One notable difference in telemedicine is transparently and proactively disclosing information about the unique features of telemedicine from two lenses: risks and benefits along with limitations of the technology.[21] Focusing on the limitations of technology is of utmost importance given the "digital divide" and unreadiness of patients who are Medicare-eligible.[22]

Advances in informed consent range from digital informed consent to the reasonable-patient standard. Given the complexity of telemedicine, a brief discussion of the reasonable-patient standard is warranted. Nearly one-half of the states in the United States have adopted this standard. In brief, the reasonable-patient standard approaches the informed consent process from the lens of the patient, not the provider or provider organization. The following elements are part and parcel of this type of informed consent: risks, benefits, and alternatives to proposed diagnostics and/or treatments. The goal is to promote shared decision-making.[16]

Informed Consent: A Focus on Sleep Telemedicine

The Position Paper for the Use of Telemedicine for the Diagnosis and Treatment of Sleep Disorders[1] clearly states that special informed consent for telemedicine encounters be drafted and that such informed consent be documented. Specifically, this Position Paper states the following regarding informed consent when utilizing asynchronous care:

"Special consent may be required when physical examination is not performed, and informed consent from the patient should include the understanding that the patient is aware of the limitation of this approach" (p. 1190).

Fields echoed the documentation of informed consent in 2020 in his paper titled "Regulatory, Legal, and Ethical Considerations of Telemedicine" published in *Sleep Medicine Clinics*.

Unique risks to telemedicine in contrast with in-person care include cyberattacks, data breaches, and privacy concerns related to who else may be at the patient's site of care.[23] Other risks may also include patient safety with regard to patient's driving during the telemedicine visit.

CLINICAL VIGNETTE

A 37-year-old female attorney contacts your sleep laboratory complaining of difficulty falling asleep because of work stress. She states that this has been happening for over 4 months and that she cannot take anymore. The receptionist schedules a telemedicine visit and sends several forms via the patient's work email including the sleep laboratory's Informed Consent form, which has not been updated since the sleep laboratory first launched its telemedicine service 2 years ago.

During the initial visit on a video platform, the provider asks, *"Did you sign all of the paperwork?"* The patient responds, *"Yes."* After this initial part of the visit, the provider reviews some of the paperwork that the patient sent to the provider's personal email account. After the visit, the provider quickly documents nearly everything that took place during the visit in the electronic health record (EHR).

As depicted in the clinical vignette, several questions may have gone through your mind as you read and reflected on this vignette including the following:

- Should the patient have been given a choice about whether she wanted an in-person or telemedicine visit?
- Should the receptionist have sent the intake forms to the patient's work email?
- Should the receptionist have used the provider's personal email account?
- Should the provider have discussed the informed consent forms with the patient during the initial visit to promote patient understanding and shared decision-making?

On reflection, the patient should have been given an informed option as to whether an in-person or telemedicine visit was appropriate based on respecting the autonomy of the patient and our earlier section on suitability. The exchange of information using work and personal emails poses an unnecessary risk for cyberattacks, not to mention violating Health Insurance Portability and Accountability Act (HIPAA) standards and perhaps organizational policies. In this vignette, the provider "consented" the patient, but there was no meaningful discussion of general informed consent and the unique risks and benefits of telemedicine.

Conclusion

Telemedicine in the practice of sleep medicine is here to stay. The COVID-19 pandemic accelerated the adoption of telemedicine, and now there is increasing empirical evidence about the benefits and limitations of telemedicine. Providers should critically determine whether telemedicine is suitable for a specific patient presenting with a specific chief complaint and whether specific diagnostics and treatments can be delivered ethically, effectively, and efficiently via telemedicine in contrast with an in-person visit. Providers should also reflect on whether telemedicine is suitable for them as discussed in this chapter. In closing, patient-centered care remains a cornerstone of effective sleep medicine whether delivered in person or via telemedicine. Part and parcel of patient-centered care is respect for patient autonomy and shared decision-making, which is realized with informed consent.

References

1. Singh J, Badr MS, Diebert W, et al. American Academy of Sleep Medicine (AASM) position paper for the use of telemedicine for the diagnosis and treatment of sleep disorders. *J Clin Sleep Med.* 2015;11(10): 1187-1198.
2. Johnson, KG, Sullivan SS, Nti A, et al. The impact of the COVID-19 pandemic on sleep medicine practices. *J Clin Sleep Med.* 2021;17(1):79-87.
3. U.S. Department of Health and Human Services. *Medicare Beneficiaries' Use of Telehealth in 2020: Trends by Beneficiary Characteristics and Location.* Washington, DC: Office of the Assistant Secretary for Planning and Evaluation; December, 2021. Available at: https://aspe.hhs.gov/sites/default/files/documents/a1d5d810fe3433e18b192be42dbf2351/medicare-telehealth-report.pdf. Accessed March 1, 2024.
4. Nouri S, Khoong EC, Lyles CR, et al. Addressing equity in telemedicine for chronic disease management during the COVID-19 pandemic. *NEJM Catal.* 2020;1(3):1-13.
5. Welch BM, Harvey J, O'Connell NS, McElligott JT. Patient preferences for direct-to-consumer telemedicine services: a nationwide survey. *BMC Health Serv Res.* 2017;17(1):1-7.

6. Scott Kruse C, Karem P, Shifflett K, et al. Evaluating barriers to adopting telemedicine worldwide: a systematic review. *J Telemed Telecare.* 2018;24(1):4-12.

7. Davis FD. Perceived usefulness, perceived ease of use, and user acceptance of information technology. *MIS Q.* 1989;13(3):319-340.

8. Kamal SA, Shafiq M, Kakria P. Investigating acceptance of telemedicine services through an extended technology acceptance model (TAM). *Technol Soc.* 2020;60:101212.

9. Jacob C, Sanchez-Vazquez A, Ivory C. Understanding clinicians' adoption of mobile health tools: a qualitative review of the most used frameworks. *JMIR Mhealth Uhealth.* 2020;8(7):1-20.

10. Wosik J, Fudim M, Cameron B, et al. Telehealth transformation: COVID-19 and the rise of virtual care. *J Am Med Inform Assoc.* 2020;27(6):957-962.

11. Paruthi S. Telemedicine in pediatric sleep. *Sleep Med Clin.* 2020;15(3S):e1-e7.

12. Talal, AH, Sofikitou EM, Jaanimägi U, et al. A framework for patient-centered telemedicine: application and lessons learned from vulnerable populations. *J Biomed Inform.* 2020;112:103622.

13. Khosla S, Deak MC, Gault D, et al. Consumer sleep technology: an American Academy of Sleep Medicine Position Statement. *J Clin Sleep Med.* 2018;14(5):877-880.

14. Guillodo E, Lemey C, Simonnet M. Clinical applications of mobile health wearable-based sleep monitoring: systematic review. *JMIR Mhealth Uhealth.* 2020;8(4):1-10.

15. Hwang D, Chang JW, Benjafield AV. Effect of telemedicine education and telemonitoring on continuous positive airway pressure adherence: the Tele-OSA randomized trial. *Am J Respir Crit Care Med.* 2018; 197(1):117-126.

16. Spatz ES, Krumholz HM, Moulton BW. The new era of informed consent: getting to a reasonable patient standard through shared decision making. *JAMA.* 2016;315(19):2063-2064.

17. Epstein RM, Street RL Jr. The values and value of patient-centered care. *Ann Fam Med.* 2011;9(2):100-103.

18. Beauchamp TL, Childress JF. *Principles of Biomedical Ethics.* 8th ed. New York: Oxford University Press; 2019.

19. Barry MJ, Edgman-Levitan S. Shared decision making-pinnacle of patient-centered care. *N Engl J Med.* 2012;366(9):780-781.

20. Fields BG. Regulatory, legal, and ethical considerations of telemedicine. *Sleep Med Clin.* 2020;15(3):409-416.

21. Chaet D, Clearfield R, Sabin JE, et al. Ethical practice in telehealth and telemedicine. *J Gen Intern Med.* 2017;32(10):1136-1140.

22. Lam K, Lu AD, Shi Y, Covinsky KE. Assessing telemedicine unreadiness among older adults in the United States during the COVID-19 pandemic. *JAMA Intern Med.* 2020;180(10):1389-1391.

23. Jacobson A. The benefits and risks of telehealth services. *Risk Manage.* 2020;67(5):10-12.

CHAPTER 9

Webside Manners

Innessa Donskoy

Introduction

Telemedicine aims to deliver high-quality care that simulates in-person clinical interactions. There are many practical aspects of virtual medicine that the provider and supporting team can work together to optimize. However, a critical component is the webside manner, or virtual bedside manner, by which a provider administers care. This is demonstrated in the way a provider prepares for, executes, and concludes virtual visits. Their actions and words should be positive, intentional, and patient-centered. These behaviors instill confidence and establish a strong care relationship. A pleasant webside manner is an important, if not critical, determining factor in patient satisfaction. Provider satisfaction also increases with a good virtual bedside manner. This can combat burnout and allow for an emotionally fulfilled provider who is capable of practicing empathy and compassion.[1] Before the visit, within the virtual clinical space, and upon discharge from the encounter, there is ample opportunity for the provider to demonstrate a positive webside manner. When successfully applied, the patient, caregivers, and clinical team can feel pleased with and proud of the overall virtual care experience.

Clinic Preparation

The delivery of care involves significant preparation by the patient and provider. The patient requesting an initial consultation with a provider has often had questions or concerns regarding this complaint for some time. The patient is perhaps anxious, hopeful, or both that there will be a simple and feasible resolution to their issue during the visit. Patients enter the encounter with a great deal of expectation and trust in the provider to address their needs. Even with in-person encounters in a medical center, this is a high bar set for the provider. Aside from simply having their clinical issue addressed, the patient's satisfaction is largely influenced by the provider's "bedside manner," the simple way in which one human relates to another in the context of the patient-provider relationship. There is much about this interaction that transcends history taking, physical examination, diagnosis, and treatment discussion. The in-person visit includes "body language, [a] rush of emotions, physical proximity, and touch."[1] This expectation is brought to the virtual visit as well. Good webside manner will creatively meet and possibly exceed these expectations, allowing the patient to come away from the encounter feeling satisfied.

PROVIDER PERSPECTIVE

The provider's demonstration of a good webside manner begins long before the specific telemedicine encounter commences. The way the provider prepares the surroundings, lighting, clothing, frame of mind, and demeanor helps portray a professional, yet warm and open time and space available to the patient. Although some providers practice telemedicine from their offices with built-in professional-looking furniture, bookshelves, and ambient lighting befitting the traditional "doctor's office" and the provider wearing a white coat,[1] the coronavirus disease 2019

(COVID-19) pandemic demonstrated that in a moment's notice, a doctor's home might become a working headquarters, with an array of personal paraphernalia and adorable interlopers. Although there is more understanding when a provider's personal life interrupts the visit,[2] ideally this should be minimized. Patient expectations about duration, quality, and often insurance-requested compensation are not different for an in-person versus a virtual visit. The service received should meet those expectations. Uninterrupted clinical time should be ensured. The door should be closed to preserve the patient's privacy and the provider's illusion of physically being in the clinic. This starts with what might seem superficial: the physical first impression. The provider's background should be clean and organized, and it should appear professional. Given that these high standards are not always possible to achieve, a neutral and non-distracting background,[3,4] whether digital or physical, can more than suffice. The lighting in the room should be bright and illuminate the provider's face.[4,5] Placement of a light fixture or a large window behind the computer screen can create this effect. The head and upper torso of the provider should be in clear view. The provider's attire and grooming should meet the high standards of an in-office appearance. This allows the patient to see the provider clearly and fosters confidence. This preparation places the provider in the clinical frame of mind. This emphasis on appearance minimizes distractions and allows for both the provider and patient to focus on the content of the visit. In this digital age, being reachable through a variety of electronic means is both a blessing and a curse as well as a new source of distraction. Minimizing the tabs of email, messaging, medical charting, ongoing projects, and other electronic documents is not enough; they must be closed. Aside from emergent matters, the provider should be wholly focused on the patient in the virtual clinic room.[3] This is when the techniques that sleep practitioners preach for relaxation in the setting of insomnia apply. Deep breathing, guided imagery, and mindfulness can help with preparing patients for sleep as well as support a provider in developing a clear and focused mindset for a smooth clinical day. At the beginning of the visit, the provider must introduce himself or herself by name and role along with anyone else who might be on the telemedicine session (other caregivers, translators, trainees).

PREVENTING BURN OUT

Being involved in the medical field already carries the risk of emotional and physical burnout. This is considerably more pronounced with telemedicine when providers are isolated from their patients, work teams, and colleagues. During a global pandemic, when support networks also become unavailable, striking a crucial work-life balance is even more challenging. In such high-stress situations, schedules and daily routines are altered, leading more individuals to seek help for sleep issues. The efficiency and lack of commute with telehealth allow sleep providers to take on additional patients, increasing provider workload. The downtime afforded by the walk between clinic rooms and offices is now replaced with sitting in a singular, hopefully comfortable, chair for most of the workday, perhaps even unconsciously forgoing meals or bathroom breaks. These are not only simple luxuries that help a provider unwind throughout the day; they are crucial moments to press "reset" and to prepare for the next patient with a clear mind and an open heart. Between patients, providers should take a few minutes to stand, stretch, look outside the window, get water or a snack, use the restroom, or simply decompress. Planning these pauses can help ensure an appropriate disassociation between work and home life, allowing the provider to thrive in both areas. The human element of this side of care must not be overlooked. Everyone benefits from a rested and recharged provider[2,3] who can hear clearly and help wholly with no distraction, exogenous or endogenous.

PATIENT PERSPECTIVE

A favorable webside manner demonstrated by the patient will also enhance the quality of a virtual visit. Just as with the provider, this starts with preparation. Upon scheduling, the care team should

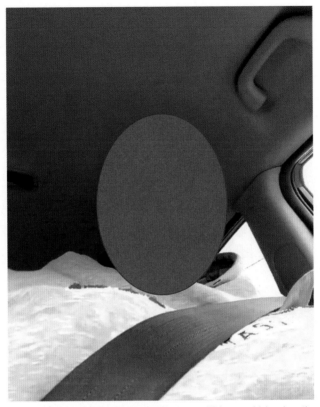

Figure 9.1 A telemedicine visit must be safe. This patient was driving a vehicle when the visit started and was asked to find a safe location.

communicate expectations for the visit as well as some suggestions, such as providing appropriate lighting, ensuring a private and safe setting, and minimizing distractions. The patient's device should be ready for the virtual visit with all other tabs closed and ancillary electronics put away. Although cliché, telemedicine allows for care at the push of a button, which can, unfortunately, lead to unsafe practices such as driving or cooking, or being in a place where privacy is not available while on the video call (see Figures 9.1 and 9.2). A video visit should not proceed if safety and privacy are not guaranteed. The patient should plan to be available and fully engaged for the entire duration of the visit. The more invested patients are in the virtual care experience, the more the provider will be able to reciprocate, leading to a pleasant and productive visit.

In the Room

The flow of a virtual visit differs from an in-person one. The waiting room no longer exists. No one collects vitals or encourages patients to wait and relax if the provider is running behind. There are no forms handed out with intake questionnaires or sleep logs to be reviewed.[3] In response, many practices have partnered with their electronic medical record (EMR) providers to develop application-based intake links and forms. These electronically collected questionnaires improve upon paper forms as they are storable, searchable, and easily tracked for progress. These EMR-based applications also utilize a check-in process to collect data about past

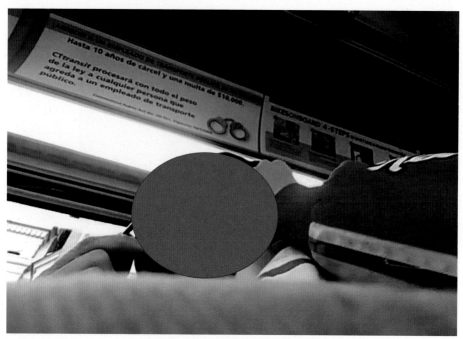

Figure 9.2 Privacy must be ensured. This patient was on a public bus when the visit started. The visit was rescheduled.

medical and surgical history, medications, and allergies. However, these are all impersonal touches. The practitioner is the first individual that the patient encounters as they click into the room. They are the greeter, medical assistant, provider, and nurse all in one. The first impression is critical to establishing a relationship and positive rapport for the remainder of the visit. Upon first glance, the provider should lean in, smile, and warmly greet the patient.[4] With the element of touch entirely removed, there is no handshake, high five, or even a fist bump to create a friendly and inviting atmosphere.[6] Body language cues can take the place of touch, and the voice can be used as an "instrument of healing,"[7] serving as an invitation to collaborate and explore the patient's concerns.

BODY LANGUAGE: PROVIDER

Although *telemedicine* refers to several remote technologies, the gold standard of replicating an in-person encounter is a real-time two-way video visit.[8] This allows body language to be part of the communication between the patient and provider. The provider's posture, voice intonation, and facial expression can show interest, care, and attentiveness.[8] Lack thereof can do the opposite. Eye contact can be challenging with virtual visits. By default, the provider looks at the center of the screen, specifically at the patient's face.[3,5] However, most computer cameras are located above the screen. For the patient, this can create the illusion of a provider looking down, appearing distracted, or appearing disinterested. The provider must balance simulating eye contact and looking at the patient on the screen. This can be accomplished by slightly minimizing the window with the patient's face and moving it closer to the top center of the screen, allowing the provider's eyes to be directed closer to the actual camera. This enables the provider to appear open-eyed and engaged.

Although the provider always must balance documentation and engagement with the patient, the virtual visit also requires utilizing one's hands to make more pronounced expressions of surprise, joy, shock, or sadness. Using motions in place of physical proximity helps connect across a two-dimensional screen. This brings out the theatrical element of the "art" of medicine, but these little gestures go a long way. Holding a patient's hand or passing a tissue in a time of distress must now be replaced with something equally impactful. A deep shrug of the shoulders or a more pronounced sigh can be powerful in demonstrating disbelief and sympathy. There is also a tremendous value in the "I wish" statement,[4] acknowledging the tangible gaps in non-verbal communication created by telemedicine and verbalizing a desire to be together.[3,4] When all else fails, sharing in the frustration of some of the challenges of telemedicine can create "social connectedness with physical distancing."[9]

BODY LANGUAGE: PATIENT

Displaying positive and professional non-verbal cues is in the control of the provider. Just as cognizant as one needs to be in demonstrating appropriate body language, the provider also must be attuned to reading the body cues of the patient across the screen. Patients are at home, comfortable, and can present more of their true selves. This should be embraced, as a comfortable patient will be more forthcoming.[10] This goes beyond what they say. A crossed-arms posture, lack of eye contact, sighing, or repeatedly checking the phone shows disengagement and possible disillusionment with the virtual visit. In pediatric and adolescent cases, in which a parent or caregiver provides most of the history, lack of age-appropriate participation from the patient can also be a red flag. One of the biggest concerns reported by patients utilizing telehealth is their skepticism regarding building a strong therapeutic bond.[2] Recognition and response to negative body language cues can be challenging but are important to fostering the patient-provider relationship.[7] Sensitively commenting on posture or lack of engagement can demonstrate the provider's attention to detail and commitment to excellent care. This honest exchange can be the turning point in a visit. On the other hand, eye contact, nodding, smiling, and an open-arms posture demonstrate engagement in the visit, increasing the likelihood of a correct diagnosis and appropriate treatment.

VERBAL COMMUNICATION

Although conducting clinic visits on camera may be a relatively new concept for sleep medicine providers, having clinical discussions is familiar territory. However, utilizing technology to take histories and plan clinical management poses unique challenges. Being aware of these differences and adjusting to them will enhance the provider's webside manner and allow for less frustrating and more fruitful exchanges. Ask the patient for permission (which is documented) if screenshots will be taken (e.g., during an upper airway examination). Patient dissatisfaction with virtual care arises from feeling that the provider did not "listen to what you had to say." Avoiding this is key. Telehealth carries a risk of technical issues, potentially leaving the patient feeling unheard. Poor signal, device malfunction, and power failure are just some examples. Providers should have a strong Internet signal, a high-speed modem and router, a direct connection to the modem if possible, updated hardware and software, and should consider a backup generator if the care they provide is emergent. Beyond technological delays, providers have been shown to speak more during virtual visits compared with in-person visits,[7] leaving less time for patient input. Silence can be uncomfortable, so providers fill it with information. Although this imparted knowledge may be helpful, it does little for relationship building or for giving patients time to process and formulate their own questions. Slower speech with ample pauses between statements allows for a reflection period and accommodates for any connection interruptions.[3,4] Providers are accustomed to validating patients' concerns during in-person visits with short, non-interrupting verbal cues, such as "mmm-hmm" or "wow." However, in a virtual setting, these add little to the encounter and risk the patient feeling interrupted, especially given the occasional connection delays.[4] Providers should allow patients to conclude their remarks and then respond with verbal reflection, summarizing what the patient shared and following with a question or emotional response.[7,8] Active listening and empathic communication are critical components for fostering a strong patient-provider relationship. When these tenets are applied in virtual care, the trust built can overcome Internet connection lapses and transcend the physical divide.

Discharge Planning

The provider is not only the first face and voice the patient encounters in the virtual visit, they are also the last. No longer does a nurse print out discharge instructions, circle new changes, or ask the patient about any further concerns. There is no front desk staff to pleasantly wave goodbye, make follow-up appointments, and engage in friendly banter with the patient. Patients simply click out of the encounter. Although there is interoffice variability on how discharge information is provided and follow-up visits are coordinated, this will likely be accomplished remotely as well, whether by video, phone, or text message. This carries a risk of the patient feeling isolated and anxious after the visit. Hope and encouragement attained from even the most uplifting visit can fade away as the patient must now navigate the medical system alone. For patients who are not accustomed to technology, this adds a great deal of stress. The provider should consider the patient's perspective, recognizing that care continues well after the virtual encounter. In concluding the visit, the provider should inquire "what" questions remain on the patient's mind, rather than "if" they have questions at all, normalizing having outstanding concerns and making sure to address them. This is also the time to go over the plan once more, reassuring the patient that it will be in the discharge instructions and describing where and how to access them. The provider should also describe in detail what patients can anticipate after the visit, clarifying if they will receive a phone call, message through the EMR, a prescription, or an order for testing that they must schedule themselves. The benefits of telehealth should be highlighted for the patient as well. Patients can now reach out to their medical teams with questions or updates utilizing messaging services embedded in the virtual care software. This can be notably more convenient than waiting on hold with the traditional call center. Providers must embrace their new role of clinical navigators as the patient exits the virtual clinic room to take the next steps independently.

The end of the visit is also the time to ask for some feedback about the virtual care experience,[3] prioritizing patient satisfaction. When this inquiry is made directly by the provider in the moment, rather than with an anonymous survey or by support staff after the fact, it demonstrates that patient satisfaction is a priority.

In concluding the encounter, the provider should thank the patient for choosing this particular care team, being open to virtual care, and dealing with the challenges of technology during the visit.[4] This highlights the patient's autonomy in selecting providers and media through which to receive care, even during a pandemic. Patients gave their time and were vulnerable enough to share private medical information. Demonstrating gratitude is often overlooked, yet what is a provider without patients to care for? These small gestures and phrases in the final moments of an encounter leave a lasting impression and showcase the visit and entire virtual care experience in a positive light.

Conclusion

Good webside manner is subjective. Some patients prefer a specific personality in their provider, more emotional versus stoic, informative versus collaborative, and so on. However, there are some fundamentals of providing virtual care that, when implemented before, during, and after a visit, reliably lead to greater patient and provider satisfaction. Providers must set aside a protected time and space for virtual encounters. They should work to eliminate any distractions whether on the screen, in the room, or internally. Providers should also be proactive in minimizing the risk of burnout with telemedicine, as they can feel isolated from colleagues while simultaneously ever available to patients. Being cognizant of the patient's and one's own body language and verbal cues will optimize communication throughout the visit. The technology utilized must be dependable. Willingness to accept feedback, show gratitude, and "hold the patient's hand" in following through with the plan will conclude the visit on a strong note and allow the patient-provider relationship to become even stronger. Whether a visit is virtual or in person, applying these concepts can enhance the interaction, which is the very purpose of having a praiseworthy "manner." When applied to telemedicine, a provider with a good webside manner will demonstrate "telecompetence,"[7] enhancing the patient's experience, enhancing their own experience, and surpassing expectations of what virtual care can achieve.[11]

References

1. Chwistek M. "Are you wearing your white coat?": Telemedicine in the time of pandemic. *JAMA*. 2020;324(2):149-150.
2. Shachak A, Alkureishi MA. Virtual care: a "Zoombie" apocalypse? *J Am Med Inform Assoc*. 2020;27(11): 1813-1815.
3. Begasse de Dhaem O, Bernstein C. Headache virtual visit toolbox: the transition from bedside manners to webside manners. *Headache*. 2020;60(8):1743-1746.
4. Chua IS, Jackson V, Kamdar M. Webside manner during the Covid-19 pandemic: maintaining human connection during virtual visits. *J Palliat Med*. 2020;23(11):1507-1509.
5. Teichert E. At the "webside." *Mod Healthc*. 2016;46(35):16-18.
6. Kelly MA, Gormley GJ. In, but out of touch: connecting with patients during the virtual visit. *Ann Fam Med*. 2020;18(5):461-462.
7. Modic MB, Neuendorf K, Windover AK. Enhancing your webside manner: optimizing opportunities for relationship-centered care in virtual visits. *J Patient Exp*. 2020;7(6):869-877.
8. McConnochie KM. Webside manner: a key to high-quality primary care telemedicine for all. *Telemed J E Health*. 2019;25(11):1007-1011.
9. Bergman D, Bethell C, Gombojav N, et al. Physical distancing with social connectedness. *Ann Fam Med*. 2020;18(3):272-277.
10. Fry E. *Doctors Work on "Webside Manner" As Telemedicine Becomes More Popular*. Fortune.com; November 2016:1. Available at: https://fortune.com/2016/11/02/telemedicine-virtual-health/. Accessed March 1, 2024.
11. Elliott T, Matsui EC, Cahill A, Smith L, Leibner L. Conducting a Professional Telemedicine Visit Using High-Quality Webside Manner. *Curr Allergy Asthma Rep*. 2022;22(2):7-12.

CHAPTER **10**

Leveraging Electronic Communications

Sreelatha Naik ▪ Anne Marie Morse

Digital health solutions (DHS) or *telehealth* refers to the broad range of synchronous and asynchronous tools that can be used for various patient needs, including but not limited to video visits, symptom tracking, or unscheduled check-ins. Digital health for sleep is not a new concept. In fact, the American Academy of Sleep Medicine (AASM) provided an overview of telemedicine use in sleep medicine in their position paper in 2015.[1] Despite this, telehealth use had been stagnated by poor reimbursement, workflow disruption, disparities in access, and lack of exposure and training, leading to poor adoption. It was not until 2020 when the coronavirus disease 2019 (COVID-19) global pandemic necessitated acceleration and expansion of "real world" implementation of various DHS across medicine. This resulted in a 300-fold increase in telemedicine visits in the United States, despite the total number of visits declining in 2020.[2] With the rapid increase in the number of televisits, it is important to consider how to best operationalize telehealth to mirror the feel of in-person visits but optimize the experience and efficiency via digital transformation.

This chapter discusses the utilization of synchronous and asynchronous electronic communication to enhance the telemedicine experience. Asynchronous communications are typically unscheduled patient- or physician-prompted interactions to elicit information about a patient's symptoms or status and may include but is not limited to questionnaires; pre-visits, post-visits, or in-between visits; patient-elected communications; or symptom tracker uploads. Synchronous communications are pre-scheduled person-to-person contacts and may include visit check-in, clinician-to-patient communication of instructions, appointment and testing scheduling, and patient communication with the clinical team. A general workflow is outlined in Figure 10.1.

In addition to the DHS for the patient-provider dyad, an additional key stakeholder to consider in sleep medicine care is the durable medical equipment (DME) provider, particularly for patients utilizing positive airway pressure (PAP) therapy. Electronic communications within cloud systems are pre-existing digital health tools that should be considered and incorporated into patient care workflows. Finally, this chapter will also discuss disparities that these communications may create for certain individuals, who may then need an alternate means of access and support.

Patient Expectations

In developing a workflow for telemedicine visits, it is important to create a process that will align with both the clinical needs and the patient's expectations and abilities. A 2005 survey of patients after the second severe acute respiratory syndrome (SARS) outbreak indicated that the majority of patients in that era reported a desire to use telehealth for their health care experience.[3] In addition, patients specified the various tools that they wanted to utilize via telemedicine (Table 10.1). Among patients who attended a sleep medicine clinic, the majority of patients reported that they already utilize both phone and email to communicate with their physician, and 63% also reported great comfort and willingness in utilizing video telemedicine.[4]

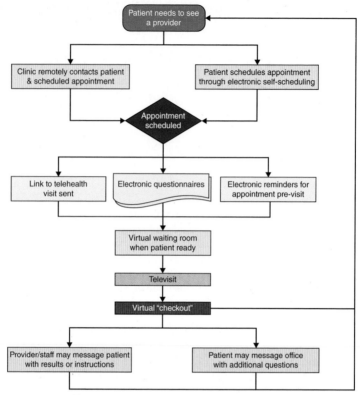

Figure 10.1   Typical workflow of telemedicine visits.

TABLE 10.1 ■ **Survey of 711 Patients Who Reported Using Internet Themselves for Health Care[3]**

Patient Desired Web-Based Experience	Percent of Patients Interested (%)
Learn about their health through educational materials	84
Review the status of their appointments	83
Send feedback to the hospital	77
Access screening tools	77
Renew prescriptions	75
Consult regarding non-urgent matters	75
Access test results	75
Had accessed the Internet to search for health information	68
Interested in long-term web-based communication	75

In a survey of families of hospitalized children on perceptions of telemedicine, 90% of respondents wanted to utilize telemedicine for consultation with a physician in case of an emergency, 90% wanted to schedule appointments, and 93% wanted to use it to communicate results from the hospital. Most respondents also felt it saved both time (88%) and money (85%).[5] Specifically, patients utilizing telemedicine in sleep medicine reported a positive impact on their access to care due to reduced travel time and cost. In addition, patients reported feeling comforted knowing that their sleep providers had the capacity for remote wireless monitoring of PAP devices and remote device control.[6]

Patient convenience is a driver for acceptance of telemedicine. With that said, from the standpoint of patient experience, it is important that televisits are able to provide easier access (in terms of time to get to an appointment), greater control of scheduling, and greater ease of exchanging information before, during, and after a visit.

Pre-visit

Patient portal systems have created a space for initiating virtual interactions including appointment scheduling (to initiate in-person visits or telemedicine appointments), pre-visit "check-ins" prior to visits, or sending messages to staff. A U.S. Department of Health and Human Services survey in 2017 showed that about 52% of Americans had access to portal systems, and 28% of them actively viewed records on such systems.[7] This data brief also notes that the percent of Americans enrolled in health portal systems increased by 24% compared with the prior survey from 2014. A systematic review assessing portal use in the in-patient setting also found that some but not all studies showed that patient portals increased patient engagement. They also increased patient safety, adherence to therapy, and patient-provider communication, but no difference was noted in objective patient health outcomes during the admission.[8]

Electronic self-scheduling of out-patient appointments via portal systems may be one means of leveraging electronic communication to enhance patient access. A meta-analysis from 2017 of 36 studies from various countries demonstrated that web-based self-scheduling of appointments resulted in a decreased no-show rate, decreased staff labor, decreased wait time, and improved satisfaction.[9] A 2021 study in the primary care setting also showed that self-scheduling of appointments may reduce inefficiencies in patient- or family-initiated schedule changes (such as canceling and rescheduling), reduce staff time, provide the convenience of scheduling outside of normal business hours, and is non-inferior to usual scheduling models in the number of no-show rates.[10]

Once an appointment is scheduled, electronic reminders may be sent via text messaging, email, or portal systems as confirmation or reminders. Text message reminders may enhance adherence to scheduled appointment times and may be preferred over telephone reminders.[11,12] Use of the patient's primary language in text messages also appears to be preferred, independent of ability to read, write, or speak English.[13]

During pre-visit check-ins, platforms may allow for review of updated insurance information, contact information, and medication list. They may also allow for completion of questionnaires, which are often used by clinicians in sleep medicine. Electronic questionnaires are discussed later in this chapter.

Virtual waiting rooms prior to interaction with the clinician may be of two types; the first type is designed for in-person visits in which a patient may be checking in from their car or outside the clinic setting to notify the office of their arrival, whereas the second type is designed for telemedicine visits, so the patient may wait in a "virtual room" for the clinical team. Education provided in waiting rooms during traditional in-person visits has been shown to improve both the waiting room experience and patients' and families' knowledge about their health.[6,14-16] Virtual waiting rooms can also be used similarly to enhance patient education about their health or about health services available at a center.

ELECTRONIC QUESTIONNAIRES

Questionnaires are an important part of information gathering in sleep medicine, which can be completed asynchronously. They can help qualify the presence of sleep disturbance and quantify

TABLE 10.2 ■ Commonly Used Questionnaires in Sleep Medicine

Questionnaire	Number of Questions	Interpretation/Value of Questionnaire
Berlin Questionnaire	10	Patients are categorized into "high risk" or "low risk" for sleep apnea groups
Epworth Sleepiness Scale (ESS)	8	Higher score implies greater sleepiness
Functional Outcomes of Sleep Questionnaire (FOSQ)	10	Higher score implies higher functioning
Insomnia Severity Index (ISI)	7	Higher score predicts greater impact of insomnia
International Restless Legs Scale (IRLS)	10	Higher score implies high burden of restless legs syndrome
Morningness-Eveningness Questionnaire	19	Helps predict circadian phase tendency
Pittsburgh Sleep Quality Index	10	Score distinguishes "good sleepers" from "bad sleepers"
Restless Legs Syndrome Quality of Life Questionnaire	18	Lower scores indicate lower quality of life
Sleep Apnea Quality of Life Index (SAQLI)	35	Reviews impact of sleep apnea as well as treatment on quality of life
Sleep Timing Questionnaire	18	Estimates habitual bedtimes
Stop-BANG	10	Stratifies patients into low, medium, or high risk for sleep apnea

the severity of any present abnormality, such as daytime sleepiness, insomnia, or restless legs syndrome. They can also help longitudinally monitor for symptom improvement or deterioration after a clinical intervention. This creates the potential for layering in machine learning and artificial intelligence models to improve diagnosis and management practices. Commonly used questionnaires in sleep medicine are shown in Table 10.2. Many of these questionnaires are available free of charge when used with permission of the creators. Some questionnaires, such as the Beck Depression Inventory, are not necessarily sleep medicine–related questionnaires, but they may be used in the sleep clinic to evaluate other disorders that may affect sleep, such as depression.

Questionnaires can be sent via portal as a text within a message to the patient prior to a visit. However, many electronic medical record systems have the ability to collect questionnaire data into a tabular form that can be integrated directly into the patient's chart. Electronic questionnaires are used both prior to telemedicine visits and also to help gather information prior to in-person visits.

Additional efforts utilizing asynchronous delivery of questionnaires and educational materials have been explored with attempts to meet the patient where it is most convenient. For example, Wake Up and Learn is a school-based sleep education and sleep disorder screening program that provides universal availability to all 7th to 12th graders.[17] The results of this program have demonstrated the ability to screen 97% of students, identifying pathological sleep features in 60% and presence of excessive daytime sleepiness in 20% of students.[18] Consideration for similar infrastructure could be proposed for work environments or in collaboration with insurance carriers.

Use of electronic questionnaires prior to the visit reinforces to patients the ease of communication. Key factors influencing whether patients will use electronic questionnaires prior to the visit include ease of completion without additional knowledge or skills, perception that questionnaires are a priority and responsibility for patients, use could lead to more efficient and personalized care, completion can be performed at the patient's convenience, and patient reminders can optimize uptake and completion.[19] Major barriers to completion of electronic questionnaires include concerns for data security, perceived usefulness of questionnaire data, stress of completing it accurately on time, competing priorities, and preferences to complete the questionnaires on other devices.[19]

The Visit

The telemedicine visit is most commonly delivered via a live interactive encounter using audio and visual capabilities for the patient and provider visit. This type of encounter can occur with the patient either at a remote clinic site, from the patient's home, or at another chosen location that is safe and private to conduct the visit. Use of a remote clinic site may be useful for patients with poor or no Internet access, those who require assistance during the visit, or for acquisition of vital signs or auscultation.

The length and complexity of medical decision-making during the visit can be heavily influenced by the digital health capabilities' pre-visit and in-between visits. For instance, one prospective study in pre-surgical patients showed that utilization of pre-visit electronic questionnaires reduced consultation time (from 25 to 12 minutes) without compromising quality or patient satisfaction relative to in-person intake of information.[20] Additional information gathering, as described later, may better inform the provider on how to personalize care for the patient.

Post-visit

An after-visit summary (AVS), delivered electronically after a visit, can be a useful tool in ensuring communication of treatment plans. Prior to the use of the AVS, research has shown that 29% to 72% of information discussed during visits is lost almost immediately, and almost one-half of the information recalled by patients is incorrect.[21] In a study evaluating AVS in the primary care setting, 82.8% of patients recalled receiving an AVS, 45.9% consulted it more than once, and 31.6 shared the AVS.[22] In patients who recalled receiving personalized free-text instruction, 96% found them to be easy to understand, and 94.4% found them to be useful.[22] Personalizing AVS formats for individual specialties and practices may be a challenge due to limitations in electronic medical record systems.[23] Patients view AVSs as useful for sharing with their family or clinicians, even if they have access to portal systems.[24]

In a study of over 5000 patients using web portals, 76.52% were aware that the AVS was available through the patient portal, and 54.71% of those patients accessed the AVS within 5 days of the office visit.[25] Patients who accessed the electronic AVS had greater interaction with the portal. Strongest beliefs associated with use of an electronic AVS were patient desire to track visits and tests and the need for accessible medical information. AVSs, sent electronically, may be a key part of reinforcing treatment plans and health education.

Electronic Communication and Cloud-Based Systems for Positive Airway Pressure Therapy

Cloud-based electronic monitoring systems have been available for leading manufacturers of PAP therapies, enhancing the care of patients with sleep apnea and also those with chronic respiratory failure requiring non-invasive or invasive mechanical ventilation. These systems allow for monitoring adherence, mask leaks, and treatment efficacy including evaluation of the apnea-hypopnea index with sub-stratification of obstructive and central events. Particularly for more advanced devices, some systems have the ability to provide breath-to-breath data, respiratory rate, tidal volumes, minute ventilation, inspiratory time, and patients' ability to trigger and cycle respiration.

Electronic monitoring of PAP data by the physician care team with electronic feedback to patients via an adherence app or device application may improve treatment adherence.[26] Monitoring patients longitudinally, even after an initial period of adherence via wireless monitoring, is important because PAP usage may vary over time after their initial experience.[27] In sleep medicine, providers may use cloud information to order device or mask-interface changes. Third-party DME providers may interface with patients on these applications to make adjustments and change settings. Cloud-based systems have areas for documentation by DME providers and means to alert the clinical team to difficulties encountered. Communication via electronic clouds systems may enhance coordination of care when there are many stakeholders involved, although greater awareness and more data about their impact on patient outcomes are needed.

In-Between Visits

Asynchronous communications in-between visits can enhance patient experience and satisfaction, but a system must be in place to be able to handle these volumes and assure responsiveness. Electronic access may mean the patient has on-demand care irrespective of the time of day. These communications more typically represent the patient contacting the provider with concerns or updates but could also take the form of provider-initiated or automated communications to obtain updates from or to educate the patient. Asynchronous information helps provide a complete clinical picture for the provider, allowing them to understand the patient's diagnosis and lead to more favorable outcomes. Chronic care management codes offer opportunity to have these services reimbursed.[28]

Telemedicine and Health Care Disparities

Although technology may help provide greater access to resource-poor areas, telemedicine alone may also introduce disparities in care. Patient surveys have demonstrated that younger age, higher education, and English as a first language were predictors of patients' interest in using Internet health resources.[3] Those living in neighborhoods with poor Internet access may not be able to choose telehealth resources as readily.[29] Having telemedicine-only resources may lead to poor access for these particular populations who may not have ready access to telemedicine-capable devices or high-speed Internet, or for those who may have poor technology literacy. As cited earlier, patients may also prefer to receive reminders in their primary language regardless of their degree of proficiency in English.

A study of AVS use in the primary care setting highlights the limitations of the AVS in individuals with limited health literacy and limited English proficiency. Individuals with limited English proficiency were more likely to "look at" (OR, 1.68; 95% CI, 1.07–2.62) and "look at and share" (OR, 1.65; 95% CI, 1.02–2.66) the AVS but were less likely to find it useful (OR, 0.68; 95% CI, 0.47–0.98) compared with English speakers.[30] Patients with limited health literacy were less likely to "look at" (OR, 0.60; 95% CI, 0.39–0.93) the AVS and less likely to find the AVS useful (OR, 0.67; 95% CI, 0.46–0.99) compared with those with adequate health literacy.[30]

In creating a workflow for telemedicine and asynchronous electronic communications, it is important to be aware that these resources are not available and accessible to everyone equally, which could create disparities in health outcomes.

Conclusion

The concerted effort to leverage electronic communications opens up the possibility to achieve greater access, create a more informed longitudinal evaluation of the patient, and augment the opportunity for machine learning and artificial intelligence models. Sleep medicine is uniquely positioned to take advantage of these DHS, as it is well-suited for virtual delivery with little need for regular in-person evaluation. Optimized use of these resources could help narrow care gaps and provide more consistent care across the globe.

References

1. Singh J, Badr MS, Diebert W, et al. American Academy of Sleep Medicine (AASM) position paper for the use of telemedicine for the diagnosis and treatment of sleep disorders. *J Clin Sleep Med*. 2015;11(10):1187-1198.
2. Fox B, Sizemore O. As Office Visits Fall, Telehealth Takes Hold. Available at: https://epicresearch.org/articles/as-office-visits-fall-telehealth-takes-hold/. Accessed March 1, 2024.
3. Rizo CA, Lupea D, Baybourdy H, et al. What Internet services would patients like from hospitals during an epidemic? Lessons from the SARS outbreak in Toronto. *J Med Internet Res*. 2005;7(4):e46.
4. Kelly JM, Schwamm LH, Bianchi MT. Sleep telemedicine: a survey study of patient preferences. *ISRN Neurol*. 2012;2012:135329.
5. Russo L, Campagna I, Ferretti B, et al. What drives attitude towards telemedicine among families of pediatric patients? A survey. *BMC Pediatr*. 2017;17(1):21.
6. Nicosia FM, Kaul B, Totten AM, et al. Leveraging telehealth to improve access to care: a qualitative evaluation of veterans' experience with the VA TeleSleep program. *BMC Health Serv Res*. 2021;21(1):77.
7. Patel V, Johnson C. Individuals' Use of Online Medical Records and Technology for Health Needs. Available at: https://www.healthit.gov/sites/default/files/page/2018-03/HINTS-2017-Consumer-Data-Brief-3.21.18.pdf. Accessed March 1, 2024.
8. Dendere R, Slade C, Burton-Jones A, et al. Patient portals facilitating engagement with inpatient electronic medical records: a systematic review. *J Med Internet Res*. 2019;21(4):e12779.
9. Zhao P, Yoo I, Lavoie J, et al. Web-based medical appointment systems: a systematic review. *J Med Internet Res*. 2017;19(4):e134.
10. North F, Nelson EM, Majerus RJ, et al. Impact of web-based self-scheduling on finalization of well-child appointments in a primary care setting: retrospective comparison study. *JMIR Med Inform*. 2021;9(3):e23450.
11. Boksmati N, Butler-Henderson K, Anderson K, Sahama T. The effectiveness of SMS reminders on appointment attendance: a meta-analysis. *J Med Syst*. 2016;40(4):90.
12. Tofighi B, Grazioli F, Bereket S, et al. Text message reminders for improving patient appointment adherence in an office-based buprenorphine program: a feasibility study. *Am J Addict*. 2017;26(6):581-586.
13. Morse E, Mitchell S. Language-appropriate appointment reminders: assessing the communication preferences of women with limited English proficiency. *J Midwifery Womens Health*. 2016;61(5):593-598.
14. Habermehl N, Diekroger E, Lazebnik R, Kim G. Injury prevention education in the waiting room of an underserved pediatric primary care clinic. *Clin Pediatr (Phila)*. 2019;58(1):73-78.
15. Williams C, Elliott K, Gall J, Woodward-Kron R. Patient and clinician engagement with health information in the primary care waiting room: a mixed methods case study. *J Public Health Res*. 2019;8(1):1476.
16. Chan Y, Nagurka R, Richardson LD, et al. Effectiveness of stroke education in the emergency department waiting room. *J Stroke Cerebrovasc Dis*. 2010;19(3):209-215.
17. Geisinger. Wake up and Learn. Available at: https://wakeupandlearn.org/. Accessed March 1, 2024.
18. Morse A, Snyder M, Liscum D, Blessing K. Wake Up and Learn: A School Based Sleep Education and Surveillance Program. Presented at: Sleep; Virtual Conference, 2021.
19. Yamada J, Kouri A, Simard SN, Segovia SA, Gupta S. Barriers and enablers to using a patient-facing electronic questionnaire: a qualitative theoretical domains framework analysis. *J Med Internet Res*. 2020;22(10):e19474.
20. Taylor SK, Andrzejowski JC, Wiles MD, et al. A prospective observational study of the impact of an electronic questionnaire (ePAQ-PO) on the duration of nurse-led pre-operative assessment and patient satisfaction. *PLoS One*. 2018;13(10):e0205439.
21. Ley P. Satisfaction, compliance and communication. *Br J Clin Psychol*. 1982;21(Pt 4):241-254.
22. Pathak S, Summerville G, Kaplan CP, et al. Patient-reported use of the after visit summary in a primary care internal medicine practice. *J Patient Exp*. 2020;7(5):703-707.
23. Federman A, Sarzynski E, Brach C, et al. Challenges optimizing the after visit summary. *Int J Med Inform*. 2018;120:14-19.
24. Federman AD, Sanchez-Munoz A, Jandorf L, et al. Patient and clinician perspectives on the outpatient after-visit summary: a qualitative study to inform improvements in visit summary design. *J Am Med Inform Assoc*. 2017;24(e1):e61-e68.

25. Emani S, Healey M, Ting DY, et al. Awareness and use of the after-visit summary through a patient portal: evaluation of patient characteristics and an application of the theory of planned behavior. *J Med Internet Res*. 2016;18(4):e77.
26. Berry RB, Beck E, Jasko JG. Effect of cloud-based sleep coaches on positive airway pressure adherence. *J Clin Sleep Med*. 2020;16(4):553-562.
27. Naik S, Al-Halawani M, Kreinin I, Kryger M. Centers for Medicare and Medicaid Services positive airway pressure adherence criteria may limit treatment to many Medicare beneficiaries. *J Clin Sleep Med*. 2019;15(2):245-251.
28. Chronic Care Management Services. Available at: https://www.cms.gov/outreach-and-education/medicare-learning-network-mln/mlnproducts/downloads/chroniccaremanagement.pdf. Accessed March 1, 2024.
29. Reed ME, Huang J, Graetz I, et al. Patient characteristics associated with choosing a telemedicine visit vs office visit with the same primary care clinicians. *JAMA Network Open*. 2020;3:e205873.
30. Nouri SS, Pathak S, Livaudais-Toman J, et al. Use and usefulness of after-visit summaries by language and health literacy among Latinx and Chinese primary care patients. *J Health Commun*. 2020;25(8):632-639.

Online History, Physical Exam, and Management

CHAPTER 11

Sleep-Disordered Breathing

Vivian Asare

Online History

Obstructive sleep apnea (OSA) is characterized by repeated episodes of upper airway collapse, often leading to intermittent hypoxia, increased sympathetic nervous system activity, and arousals from sleep.[1,2] These physiological changes can cause daytime dysfunction such as daytime sleepiness or fatigue and the most common nocturnal symptom, snoring.[3] The approach to the online history will involve gathering a detailed history similar to that obtained at an in-person visit.[4]

SYMPTOMS

Fatigue is one of the most common presenting symptoms of OSA, and questionnaires such as the Epworth Sleepiness Scale (an 8-item scale with each item scored from 0 to 3, ranging from 0 to 24, with higher scores indicating more sleepiness)[5] can help distinguish fatigue from daytime sleepiness.[6] Soliciting whether a patient is drowsy is important, especially in assessing the risk for motor vehicle accidents with drowsy driving. In a systematic review evaluating clinical examination accuracy in diagnosing OSA,[6] a patient history endorsing nocturnal choking or gasping was the most useful (summary likelihood ratio [LR], 3.3; 95% confidence interval [CI], 2.1-4.6) when the diagnosis was established by apnea-hypopnea index (AHI ≥10/h). Snoring is common in sleep apnea patients but is not useful for establishing the diagnosis (summary LR, 1.1; 95% CI, 1.0-1.1). In this review, in community-based individuals with a body mass index (BMI) less than 26 and mild reported snoring are unlikely to have moderate or severe OSA (LR, 0.07; 95% CI, 0.03-0.19 at threshold of AHI ≥15/h).[6] Initial questions in a routine health maintenance evaluation can include questions about snoring and daytime sleepiness; positive findings should then lead to a more comprehensive sleep history. The Adult OSA Task Force of the American Academy of Sleep Medicine (AASM) lists questions that should be included in a comprehensive sleep history of a patient suspected to have OSA, including snoring, witnessed apneas, gasping/choking episodes, excessive sleepiness not explained by other factors, including assessment of sleepiness severity by the Epworth Sleepiness Scale, morning headaches, nocturia, sleep fragmentation/sleep maintenance insomnia, total sleep amount, and decreased concentration and memory.[7] In patients referred to a sleep center, snoring has been found to have high sensitivity (80%-90%), but low specificity (20%-50%) for the diagnosis of OSA, whereas nocturnal choking or gasping has a lower sensitivity (52%) but is more specific (84%).[6] A discussion of nocturia is helpful in describing sleep fragmentation, and in a population study, at least two episodes of nocturia per night were reported in 37.4% of individuals with an AHI of at least 20 per hour compared with 25.6% of those with an AHI of less than 20 per hour (adjusted odds ratio, 1.64 [95% CI, 1.03-2.55]).[8] Morning headaches are also a common presenting symptom, often described as lasting about 2 hours after awakening with unclear etiology. These chronic morning headaches are twice as likely to occur in patients with OSA as compared with the general population.[9]

RISK FACTORS

There are known risk factors associated with a higher prevalence of OSA. During a telemedicine encounter, both modifiable and unmodifiable risk factors for OSA should be discussed. Unmodifiable risk factors include age, sex, and family history. Modifiable risk factors such as obesity, medication use, and substance use (which can affect upper airway tone); comorbid conditions; and nasal congestion and overall patency should be included in the patient history and evaluation.

OSA risk increases with age and is more prevalent in males. In a study evaluating males 65 years of age and older, moderate OSA was found in 23% of males younger than 72 years of age and 30% of males older than 80 years of age.[10] Males are at higher risk for OSA than females, until menopause, when the risk becomes similar.[11] In a systematic review, at a diagnostic AHI of 5/h, the overall population prevalence of OSA ranged from 9% to 38% and was higher in males. The prevalence increased with increasing age and was as high as 90% in males and 78% in females in some older adult groups.[12] Obesity (BMI >30 kg/m^2), specifically increased waist-to-hip ratio (WHR) and neck circumference (NC), has been found to increase the risk for OSA.[13] BMI data should be reviewed and included in the history gathering of a patient being evaluated for suspected OSA.

COMORBID CONDITIONS

Certain comorbid conditions have been found to be associated with an increased incidence of OSA. A comprehensive medical history should be performed during a telemedicine encounter with the patient. These high-risk patients include individuals who are obese and individuals with a history of atrial fibrillation, refractory hypertension, type 2 diabetes, congestive heart failure, stroke, nocturnal dysrhythmias, pulmonary hypertension, or high-risk occupations (e.g., commercial truck drivers), and those being evaluated for bariatric surgery.[7] OSA has been found to be associated with as high as a 2- to 3-fold increased risk for cardiovascular and metabolic disease.[14] Patients with refractory hypertension have been found to have high prevalence of OSA. In a 2014 study, 82% of patients with refractory hypertension had OSA, and 55% had moderate/severe OSA. These patients with moderate/severe OSA were more likely to have a higher prevalence of diabetes and left ventricular hypertrophy and tended to be obese, older adults, and have a larger waist-to-neck circumference.[15] In a recent prospective cohort study, 85% of patients with atrial fibrillation were found to have OSA, and of those who were not found to have OSA, 27% had an elevated AHI during REM sleep.[16] Similarly, there is a high prevalence of OSA in up to 65% to 85% of patients with diabetes,[17] 71% to 77% of patients undergoing bariatric surgery,[18] and 71% of patients with stroke.[19]

Online Physical Examination

The physical examination can provide vital information and under normal circumstances should include cardiovascular, respiratory, neurological, and upper airway and craniofacial system evaluations.[7] In a telemedicine encounter, however, the examination will be limited and should focus on the presence of obesity, measurements of BMI and NC, and visualization of upper airway and craniofacial anatomy.

Depending on whether a patient has digital wearable devices and home monitoring systems, such as a blood pressure monitor, pulse oximeter, or a scale, a set of vital signs may be collected at the start of the visit. Body weight, BMI, and NC may also be self-measured by patients and provided to clinicians during a telemedicine encounter; these measurements have been found to correlate with both the presence and severity of OSA. These measures along with craniofacial measurements, pharyngeal scores, and tonsil size demonstrate a high positive predictive value (PPV) of 90% to 100%, but a lower negative predictive value of 49% to 89%.[20]

Naso-oropharyngeal airway examination may be difficult through video because of a lack of tools and lighting, but some assessment of tongue scalloping, jaw occlusion, dental health, and evidence of retrognathia or micrognathia may be obtainable and can inform about the risk for sleep-disordered breathing. With the patient's permission, screenshots from the display can be pasted into the electronic medical record. The following are examples of some elements of the remote physical examination that can be achieved during a remote telemedicine session.

ANTHROPOMETRIC MEASUREMENTS

Obesity plays an important role in the pathogenesis of OSA, but more specifically, in localized fat distribution. Obesity indexes such as BMI, waist circumference (WC), NC, and WHR affect the severity of OSA in different ways.[21] In a study evaluating differences between anthropometric profiles and their association with OSA, differences were found between males and females. In males, WC (p=0.035), NC (p=0.006), and WHR (p=0.003) were significantly elevated in the OSA group, whereas in females, BMI (p=0.05), WC (p=0.008), and WHR (p=0.001) were significantly higher in the OSA group. WHR consistent with central weight distribution was found to be the most reliable risk factor for OSA and highly correlated with AHI in both sexes. In males, NC showed the tightest correlation with AHI.[21] An NC >17 inches in males or >16 inches in females with a BMI $\geq$30 kg/m² are risk factors for OSA.[7,22]

TELEMEDICINE EXAMINATION IN PATIENTS SUSPECTED OF HAVING A SLEEP BREATHING DISORDER

In the initial telemedicine upper airway and craniofacial examination, observing the general shape of the patient's face while forward facing and then turning to the left and right can provide information about the presence of retrognathia or micrognathia. Retrognathia and micrognathia can cause the tongue to lie in a more posterior position and subsequently lead to obstruction of the upper airway. Mandibular deficiency syndrome, an inferiorly placed hyoid bone relative to the mandibular plane along with elongation of the soft palate, is a common abnormality that predisposes individuals to OSA due to upper airway narrowing.[23] The patient can then be asked to open their mouth and face the camera. Often there is insufficient light to visualize the posterior pharynx, soft and hard palate, uvula, and tonsils. However, the tongue may be extended out of the mouth and examined. Tongue findings that suggest crowding include ridging or scalloping of the tongue and macroglossia. Fat deposition in the tongue increases with severity of obesity, and patients with OSA are found to have more tongue fat than controls, even while controlling for BMI.[24] If sufficient lighting can be arranged to inspect the oropharynx, the pharyngeal walls, uvula, and tonsils may be evaluated. Narrowing of the upper airway by the lateral pharyngeal walls has the highest association with OSA, and the site of obstruction is most commonly at the level of the oropharynx.[25] The Mallampati score is a classification used to reflect oropharyngeal crowding on a 4-point scale and was found to predict OSA. Each point increase in the score was associated with an odds ratio of 2.5 (95% CI [1.2, 5.0]) for OSA and predicted a 5-point higher AHI (coefficient = 5.3 [0.2-10]), independent of many other physical findings and symptoms.[26] Mallampati scoring may be attempted, but it has limitations with poor lighting, as described earlier.

OVERALL IMPRESSION

Images of the patient can suggest obesity, the findings consistent with polycystic ovarian syndrome (Figures 11.1 and 11.2) and facial skeletal abnormalities.

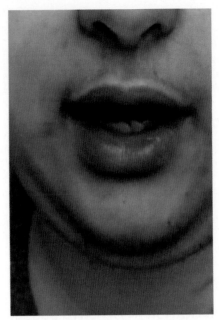

Figure 11.1   Obesity and abnormal facial hair can be noted as in this patient with polycystic ovarian syndrome.

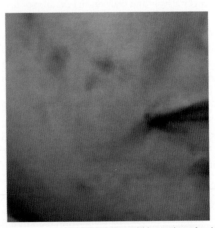

Figure 11.2   Acne can be seen during inspection that could be a sign of polycystic ovarian syndrome.

JAW AND DENTAL STRUCTURES

Since facial skeletal and dental abnormalities may be risk factors for OSA, this part of the examination is helpful (Figures 11.3 and 11.4).

Oral Examination

This might be difficult to achieve, and results will depend on the lighting and the resolution of the patient's camera (Figures 11.5 and 11.6).

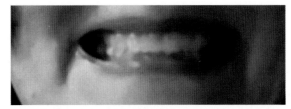

Figure 11.3 Alignment of the upper and lower teeth is an important aspect of the examination.

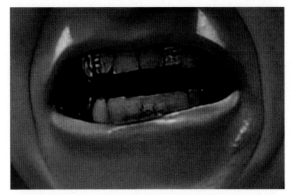

Figure 11.4 Integrity of dental structure is a key element of the examination, and an oral appliance must be considered as treatment.

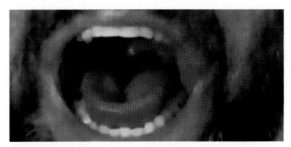

Figure 11.5 Even an out-of-focus fuzzy image can show scalloping of the tongue.

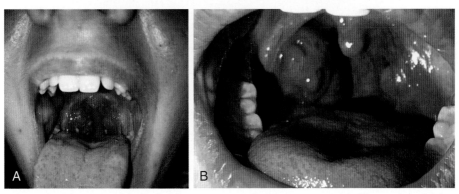

Figure 11.6 When instructing the patient to open their mouth wide and move their head to maximize lighting, examining the tonsils is possible, as in these patients with (A) tonsillar stones and (B) enlarged tonsils.

DIAGNOSTIC TESTING

Testing is indicated when there is a moderate to high risk of the patient having a sleep breathing disorder. One useful tool to assess risk is the STOP-Bang instrument. This instrument assesses the presence of: **S**noring; **T**iredness; **O**bserved apnea; high blood **P**ressure; **B**MI ≥35; **A**ge ≥50; **N**eck collar size >16 inches; **G**ender = male. Interpretation of the instrument: OSA—Low Risk: Yes to 0 to 2 questions; OSA—Intermediate Risk: Yes to 3 to 4 questions; OSA—High Risk: Yes to 5 to 8 questions.[27]

Home sleep apnea testing is the most common diagnostic procedure in suspected cases. In-laboratory testing can also be performed (see Chapter 15). Most often three or four channel systems are used (Figures 11.7 and 11.8).

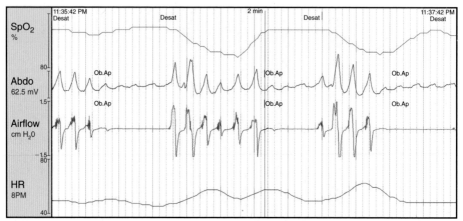

Figure 11.7   The most commonly used home sleep tests record SpO_2, effort, airflow, and heart rate. *(Figure 47.18, Kryger MH, Avidan AY, Goldstein C. Atlas of Clinical Sleep Medicine. Elsevier; 2023.)*

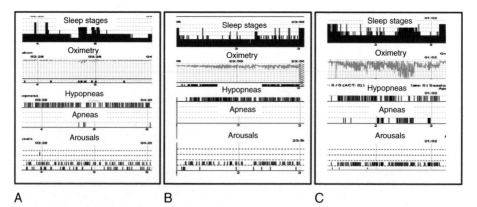

A   B   C

Figure 11.8   Results of in-laboratory polysomnography can further characterize phenotypes and inform treatment decisions. These three patients had similar apnea-hypopnea indices. **A,** This patient has many arousals but few apneas and little hypoxemia. The patients in (**B**) and (**C**) have progressively more hypoxemia.

TREATMENT

Almost all aspects of treatment (positive airway pressure [PAP] therapy, oral appliance) can be ordered electronically. Most insurance carriers require documentation of adherence to treatment (Figure 11.9). Settings can be verified and adjustments to therapy made (Figure 11.10).

FOLLOW-UP

The breathing pattern can be examined with some remote monitoring systems (Figure 11.11). The patient can obtain information about treatment efficacy smart phone apps communicating with the PAP device or with a continuously monitoring consumer-grade oximeter wearable (Figure 11.12). Data concerning abnormal breathing events, mask leak, or a continuously recording oximeter (Figure 11.13) can be transmitted to the medical practitioner who can initiate corrective steps.

Compliance report

Usage	03/20/2023 – 04/18/2023
Usage days	**30/30 days (100%)**
>= 4 hours	30 days (100%)
< 4 hours	0 days (0%)
Usage hours	248 hours 37 minutes
Average usage (total days)	8 hours 17 minutes
Average usage (days used)	8 hours 17 minutes
Median usage (days used)	8 hours 17 minutes
Total used hours (value since last reset - 04/18/2023)	5,360 hours

AirCurve 10 ASV	
Serial number	
Mode	ASVAuto
Min EPAP	10 cmH2O
Max EPAP	15 cmH2O
Min PS	4 cmH2O
Max PS	15 cmH2O

Therapy			
Leaks - L/min	Median: **0.0**	95th percentile: **18.4**	Maximum: **43.1**
Events per hour	AI: **1.4**	HI: **2.8**	AHI: **4.2**

Usage - hours

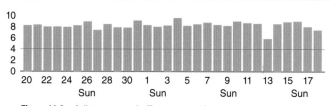

Figure 11.9 Adherence and efficacy report from a compliant patient.

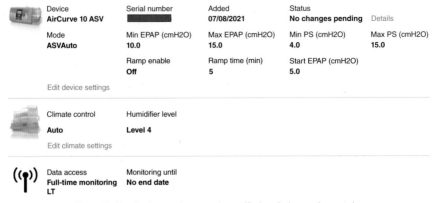

Device	Serial number	Added	Status	
AirCurve 10 ASV	▓▓▓▓	**07/08/2021**	**No changes pending**	Details
Mode	Min EPAP (cmH2O)	Max EPAP (cmH2O)	Min PS (cmH2O)	Max PS (cmH2O)
ASVAuto	**10.0**	**15.0**	**4.0**	**15.0**
	Ramp enable	Ramp time (min)	Start EPAP (cmH2O)	
	Off	**5**	**5.0**	

Edit device settings

Climate control	Humidifier level
Auto	**Level 4**

Edit climate settings

Data access	Monitoring until
Full-time monitoring	**No end date**
LT	

Figure 11.10   Device settings can be verified and changed remotely.

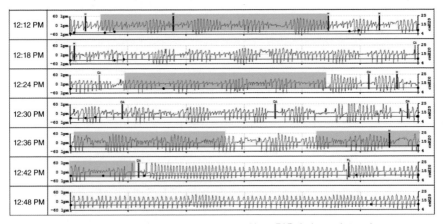

Figure 11.11   Examination of a breathing pattern as captured by a PAP device and stored on a server. *PAP,* Positive airway pressure.

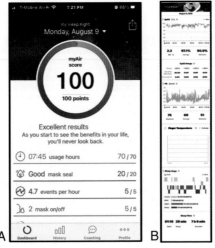

Figure 11.12   A, Data from a smart device communicating with a PAP device. **B,** Data from a continuously monitoring wearable oximeter. *PAP,* Positive airway pressure.

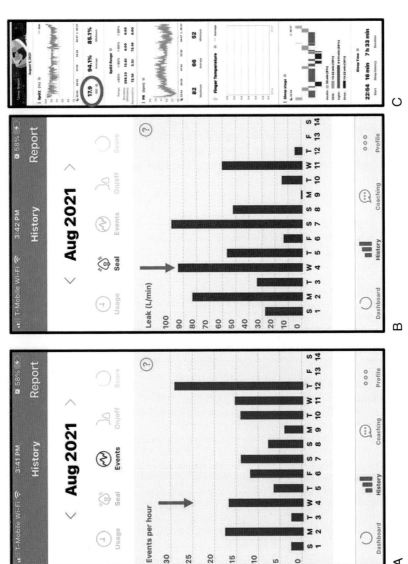

Figure 11.13 Data available to the patient. *A* and **B,** Data from a PAP machine showing nights with increased abnormal breathing events and leaks (e.g., August 4, *arrows*). **C,** The corresponding night oximeter report from the wearable. *PAP,* Positive airway pressure.

Conclusion

Telemedicine has become more widely used in ambulatory clinics worldwide due to the coronavirus disease 2019 (COVID-19) pandemic. All aspects of management can be achieved in typical uncomplicated OSA patients in a cost-effective manner.[28]

This chapter focused on the management of a patient suspected of having OSA by utilizing technology, such as a smart device, that would be widely accessible to all patient populations. A comprehensive history is still probably the strongest evidence supporting sleep-disordered breathing. Telemedicine may allow for a focused physical examination, centering around data collection such as BMI, NC, and visualizing craniofacial features and some oropharyngeal structures that have been found to predispose patients to OSA. The Adult OSA Task Force of the AASM position on telehealth prior to COVID-19 and social distancing restrictions discusses the role of a patient presenter. This would involve a distant provider assisting to perform an examination; for example, a nurse may apply an electronic stethoscope to a patient's chest so heart and lung sounds could be auscultated by the provider conducting the telemedicine consultation.[4] This approach would allow a comprehensive examination; however, limitations such as access to a patient presenter, cost to the patient, and technology and equipment operation may not always prove feasible.

References

1. Heinzer R, Vat S, Marques-Vidal P, et al. Prevalence of sleep-disordered breathing in the general population: the HypnoLaus study. *Lancet Respir Med.* 2015;3(4):310-318.
2. Kapur VK, Auckley DH, Chowdhuri S, et al. Clinical practice guideline for diagnostic testing for adult obstructive sleep apnea: an American Academy of Sleep Medicine Clinical Practice Guideline. *J Clin Sleep Med.* 2017;13(3):479-504.
3. Rundo JV. Obstructive sleep apnea basics. *Cleve Clin J Med.* 2019;86(9 suppl 1):2-9.
4. Singh J, Badr MS, Diebert W, et al. American Academy of Sleep Medicine (AASM) position paper for the use of telemedicine for the diagnosis and treatment of sleep disorders. *J Clin Sleep Med.* 2015;11(10):1187-1198.
5. Johns MW. A new method for measuring daytime sleepiness: the Epworth sleepiness scale. *Sleep.* 1991;14(6):540-545.
6. Myers KA, Mrkobrada M, Simel DL. Does this patient have obstructive sleep apnea?: The Rational Clinical Examination systematic review. *JAMA.* 2013;310(7):731-741.
7. Epstein LJ, Kristo D, Strollo PJ Jr, et al. Clinical guideline for the evaluation, management and long-term care of obstructive sleep apnea in adults. *J Clin Sleep Med.* 2009;5(3):263-276.
8. Martin SA, Appleton SL, Adams RJ, et al. Nocturia, other lower urinary tract symptoms and sleep dysfunction in a community-dwelling cohort of men. *Urology.* 2016;97:219-226.
9. Russell MB, Kristiansen HA, Kværner KJ. Headache in sleep apnea syndrome: epidemiology and pathophysiology. *Cephalalgia.* 2014;34(10):752-755.
10. Mehra R, Stone KL, Blackwell T, et al. Prevalence and correlates of sleep-disordered breathing in older men: osteoporotic fractures in men sleep study. *J Am Geriatr Soc.* 2007;55(9):1356-1364.
11. Young T, Finn L, Austin D, Peterson A. Menopausal status and sleep-disordered breathing in the Wisconsin Sleep Cohort Study. *Am J Respir Crit Care Med.* 2003;167(9):1181-1185.
12. Senaratna CV, Perret JL, Lodge CJ, et al. Prevalence of obstructive sleep apnea in the general population: a systematic review. *Sleep Med Rev.* 2017;34:70-81.
13. Young T, Shahar E, Nieto FJ, et al. Predictors of sleep-disordered breathing in community-dwelling adults. *Arch Intern Med.* 2002;162(8):893-900.
14. Gotlieb D, Punjabi NM. Diagnosis and management of obstructive sleep apnea: a review. *JAMA.* 2020;323(14):1389-1400.
15. Muxfeldt ES, Margallo VS, Guimarães GM, Salles GF. Prevalence and associated factors of obstructive sleep apnea in patients with resistant hypertension. *Am J Hypertens.* 2014;27(8):1069-1078.

16. Abumuamar AM, Dorian P, Newman D, Shapiro CM. The prevalence of obstructive sleep apnea in patients with atrial fibrillation. *Clin Cardiol*. 2018;41(5):601-607.
17. Reutrakul S, Mokhlesi B. Obstructive sleep apnea and diabetes: a state of the art review. *Chest*. 2017;152(5): 1070-1086.
18. Peromaa-Haavisto P, Tuomilehto H, Kössi J, et al. Prevalence of obstructive sleep apnoea among patients admitted for bariatric surgery: a prospective multicentre trial. *Obes Surg*. 2016;26(7):1384-1390.
19. Seiler A, Camilo M, Korostovtseva L, et al. Prevalence of sleep-disordered breathing after stroke and TIA: a meta-analysis. *Neurology*. 2019;92(7):e648-e654.
20. Kushida CA, Efron B, Guilleminault C. A predictive morphometric model for the obstructive sleep apnea syndrome. *Ann Intern Med*. 1997;127(8 Pt 1):581-587.
21. Lim YH, Choi J, Kim KR, et al. Sex-specific characteristics of anthropometry in patients with obstructive sleep apnea: neck circumference and waist-hip ratio. *Ann Otol Rhinol Laryngol*. 2014;123(7):517-523.
22. Cizza G, de Jonge L, Piaggi P, et al. Neck circumference is a predictor of metabolic syndrome and obstructive sleep apnea in short-sleeping obese men and women. *Metab Syndr Relat Disord*. 2014;12(4): 231-241.
23. Cistulli PA. Craniofacial abnormalities in obstructive sleep apnoea: implications for treatment. *Respirology*. 1996;1(3):167-174.
24. Kim AM, Keenan BT, Jackson N, et al. Tongue fat and its relationship to obstructive sleep apnea. *Sleep*. 2014;37(10):1639-1648.
25. Koren A, Groselj LD, Fajdiga I. CT comparison of primary snoring and obstructive sleep apnea syndrome: role of pharyngeal narrowing ratio and soft palate-tongue contact in awake patient. *Eur Arch Otorhinolaryngol*. 2009;266(5):727-734.
26. Nuckton TJ, Glidden DV, Browner WS, et al. Physical examination: Mallampati score as an independent predictor of obstructive sleep apnea. *Sleep*. 2006;29(7):903-908.
27. STOP-Bang Questionnaire. Available at: http://www.stopbang.ca/patient/screening.php. Accessed March 1, 2024.
28. Pumpo M, Nurchis MC, Moffa A, et al. Multiple-access versus telemedicine home-based sleep apnea testing for obstructive sleep apnea (OSA) diagnosis: a cost-minimization study. *Sleep Breath*. 2022;26(4): 1641-1647.

CHAPTER 12

Hypersomnia

Vivian Asare

Introduction

Patients with hypersomnia can be managed with telemedicine.[1,2] Hypersomnia is a major public health issue and causes detrimental effects to an individual's daytime functioning, quality of life, and overall safety. Excessive daytime sleepiness (EDS) is estimated to cause almost one-fifth of the motor vehicle accidents in the United States. Furthermore, patients with EDS have an increased risk for work-related injury, decreased workplace productivity, and overall lower quality of life.[3] Hypersomnia of central origin includes a group of disorders with the primary complaint being EDS without evidence of a disturbance of nocturnal sleep, circadian rhythm, or sleep-disordered breathing.[4] Ascertaining the severity of hypersomnolence is an important part of the history and can be performed by asking direct questions about sleepiness in various sedentary situations, such as reading, driving, working, or watching television. Utilizing questionnaires such as the Epworth Sleepiness Scale (ESS)[5] is a more standardized approach of measuring the degree of hypersomnolence propensity and allows for monitoring the response to treatment over time. In the telemedicine encounter, the history will be similar to an in-person visit; however, the physical examination will be more focused and limited and will provide vital information to help determine the cause of the presenting symptoms. In this chapter, we will discuss the different types of hypersomnia and the important questions to include in an online history. We will then conclude with a description of a focused online examination for the patient presenting with EDS.

Online History

NARCOLEPSY TYPE I AND TYPE II

Narcolepsy type I is a disorder defined by EDS and episodes of REM intrusion, such as cataplexy. Asking questions about muscle weakness triggered by intense emotions such as laughter or anger will help patients understand the sensation. Specifically, cataplexy is a brief episode (<2 minutes) of loss of symmetrically bilateral muscle tone, without loss of consciousness.[2] The defining feature between narcolepsy type I and type II is the presence of cataplexy and low cerebrospinal fluid (CSF) hypocretin concentration (<110 pg/mL) in type I narcolepsy.[2] Patients may describe having an irrepressible need to sleep and an inability to stay alert. Patients may also describe intense sudden lapses into sleep, known as *sleep attacks*. Asking questions about sleep patterns and frequency of napping is an essential part of the history. Assessing how patients feel after a nap may help distinguish narcolepsy from other forms of hypersomnolence such as idiopathic hypersomnolence. In narcoleptic patients, naps are often described as transiently refreshing. In contrast, more than two-thirds of patients with idiopathic hypersomnia describe naps as non-restorative.[6] Although a non-specific symptom, about 50% of patients with narcolepsy report sleep paralysis or hypnagogic/hypnopompic hallucinations.[7] Nighttime sleep in patients with narcolepsy is often fragmented. The onset of symptoms is usually between 10 and 25 years of age but may have a bimodal distribution, with a secondary peak in females at about 35 years of age.[6,8] Useful screeners to document severity of symptoms are available online at: https://www.narcolepsylink.com/screening-and-diagnosis/screeners/.

IDIOPATHIC HYPERSOMNIA

Idiopathic hypersomnia is characterized by EDS and prolonged sleep inertia that is not explained by another sleep disorder. *Sleep inertia* refers to significant difficulty awakening from sleep in the morning or after a nap. Patients may describe sleep drunkenness associated with mental confusion (incoherent speech, disorientation, inappropriate behaviors, amnesia) of variable duration, and this may persist several hours after arousal.[9] Asking whether a patient uses an alarm may elicit a history of sleeping through multiple alarms and having no recollection of turning them off. A clear sleep-wake history and duration of total sleep time may help provide information about unrefreshing long sleep, often more than 10 hours in patients with idiopathic hypersomnia.[10] The Idiopathic Hypersomnia Severity Scale has been developed to document the impact of the disorder. This is a 14-question instrument with each question having a score of 0 to 3. Severity is: mild (0–12); moderate (13–25); severe (26–38); very severe (39–50).

IDIOPATHIC HYPERSOMNIA SEVERITY SCALE

On the basis of your symptoms during the past month:

1. What for you is the <u>ideal duration of night-time sleep</u> *(at the weekend or on holiday, for example)?*
   - 3 ☐ 11 hours or more
   - 2 ☐ more than 9 hours and less than 11 hours
   - 1 ☐ between 7 hours and 9 hours
   - 0 ☐ less than 7 hours

2. When circumstances require that you get up at a particular time in the morning *(for example, for work or studies, or to take the children to school during the week)*, do you <u>feel that you have not</u> had enough sleep?
   - 3 ☐ always
   - 2 ☐ often
   - 1 ☐ sometimes
   - 0 ☐ never

3. Is it <u>extremely difficult</u> for you, or even <u>impossible</u>, to wake in the morning <u>without several alarm</u> calls or the help of someone close?
   - 3 ☐ always
   - 2 ☐ often
   - 1 ☐ sometimes
   - 0 ☐ never

4. After a night's sleep, how long does it take you <u>to feel you are functioning properly after you get up</u> *(in other words fully functional, both physically and intellectually)?*
   - 4 ☐ 2 hours or more
   - 3 ☐ more than 1 hour but less than 2 hours
   - 2 ☐ between 30 minutes and 1 hour
   - 1 ☐ less than 30 minutes
   - 0 ☐ I feel I am functioning properly as soon as I wake up

5. In the minutes after waking up, do you ever <u>do irrational things</u> and/or <u>say irrational things, and/or</u> <u>are you very clumsy</u> *(for example, tripping up, breaking things, or dropping things)?*
   - 3 ☐ always
   - 2 ☐ often
   - 1 ☐ sometimes
   - 0 ☐ never

6. During the day, when circumstances allow, <u>do you ever take a nap?</u>
   - 4 ☐ very often (6–7 times a week)
   - 3 ☐ often (4–5 times a week)
   - 2 ☐ sometimes (2–3 times a week)
   - 1 ☐ rarely (once a week)
   - 0 ☐ never

7. What for you is the <u>ideal length of your naps</u> *(at the weekend or on holiday, for example)?*
   ☐ *Note: If you take several naps, add them all together.*
   3 ☐ 2 hours or more
   2 ☐ more than 1 hour and less than 2 hours
   1 ☐ less than 1 hour
   0 ☐ no naps
8. In general, <u>how do you feel after a nap</u>?
   3 ☐ very sleepy
   2 ☐ sleepy
   1 ☐ awake
   0 ☐ wide awake
9. During the day, <u>while carrying out activities that are not very stimulating, do you ever</u> <u>struggle</u> to stay awake?
   4 ☐ very often (at least twice a day)
   3 ☐ often (4–7 times a week)
   2 ☐ sometimes (2–3 times a week)
   1 ☐ rarely (once a week or less)
   0 ☐ never
10. Do you consider that your hypersomnolence has <u>an impact on your general health</u> *(i.e., lack of energy, no motivation to do things, physical fatigue on exertion, decrease in physical fitness)?*
    4 ☐ very significant
    3 ☐ significant
    2 ☐ moderate
    1 ☐ minor
    0 ☐ no impact
11. Do you consider that your hypersomnolence <u>is a problem in terms of your proper</u> <u>intellectual</u> <u>functioning</u> *(i.e., problems with concentration, memory problems, decrease in your intellectual performance)?*
    4 ☐ very significant
    3 ☐ significant
    2 ☐ moderate
    1 ☐ minor
    0 ☐ no problem
12. Do you consider that your hypersomnolence <u>affects your mood</u> *(for example, sadness, anxiety, hypersensitivity, irritability)?*
    4 ☐ very severely
    3 ☐ severely
    2 ☐ moderately
    1 ☐ slightly
    0 ☐ not at all
13. Do you consider that your hypersomnolence <u>prevents you from carrying out daily tasks</u> <u>properly</u> *(family-related or household tasks, school, leisure or job-related tasks)?*
    4 ☐ very significantly
    3 ☐ significantly
    2 ☐ moderately
    1 ☐ slightly
    0 ☐ not at all
14. Do you consider that your hypersomnolence <u>is a problem in terms of your driving a car</u>?
    4 ☐ very significant
    3 ☐ significant
    2 ☐ moderate
    1 ☐ minor
    0 ☐ no problem
    ☐ I do not drive

A useful screener to document severity of IH is available for download: https://www.livingwithih.com/assets/pdf/IHSS_Patient_Download.pdf

HYPERSOMNIA DUE TO A MEDICAL DISORDER

A comprehensive medical history should be included in the telemedicine encounter of a patient being evaluated for EDS. In this disorder, a history of EDS in the setting of a major underlying medical or neurological condition is present. In the subtype of residual hypersomnolence after the treatment of obstructive sleep apnea (OSA), a patient will have a history of adequately treated OSA, with a compliant data download and effective pressure settings and yet still report daytime sleepiness. Other conditions that have been found to cause hypersomnolence include metabolic encephalopathy,[11] neurodegenerative disorders such as Parkinson disease,[12] stroke,[13] rheumatological diseases, chronic infections, head trauma, brain tumors, and cancer.[2] EDS is often an early symptom in post-stroke survivors, and the prevalence rate ranges from 18% to 72%.[9] In a recent cross-sectional study, 62% of patients with hypertension reported EDS[14]; however, the underlying medical condition should be judged as to whether it is the direct cause of hypersomnolence.[2]

HYPERSOMNIA DUE TO A PSYCHIATRIC DISORDER OR SUBSTANCE USE

Hypersomnolence is a common complaint across mood disorders, especially in major depressive disorder (MDD).[6] As part of the online history in a telemedicine visit, a comprehensive psychiatric history should be included in the patient evaluation. Hypersomnolence plays a significant role in the course of psychiatric illness and is associated with treatment resistance, increased risk for suicide, and functional impairment.[15] A patient presenting with hypersomnolence and known mood disorder may be at high risk for an exacerbation of mood symptoms. Hypersomnolence in MDD significantly varies across age, gender, and studies, ranging from 8.9% in childhood (6–13 years of age) to a high rate of 75.8% in young adulthood. The frequency of hypersomnolence in MDD was higher in females.[6] Patients with psychiatric disorders are also at risk for OSA and other sleep disorders such as narcolepsy, restless legs syndrome, insomnia, and circadian rhythm disorders. Therefore questions about symptoms of these disorders should be included in the history. A list of current medications should be reviewed, such as the use of sleep aids, benzodiazepines, anxiolytic medications, antipsychotics, antihistamines, antiepileptics (except lamotrigine), and antidepressants, as these medications may contribute to sleep disturbances or hypersomnolence.[6] Social history discussion about alcohol or recreational drugs (marijuana, opiates, barbiturates) use may also provide useful clinical information about the etiology of presenting symptoms.

INSUFFICIENT SLEEP SYNDROME

A discussion about sleep duration during the weekdays and weekends is important for a history of insufficient sleep syndrome. In this disorder, patients are likely to describe a history of curtailed sleep time due to an alarm clock or being awakened by another person, and they may sleep for longer periods when these measures are removed. Patients have complaints of EDS; however, with extended sleep time, there is resolution of symptoms. A sleep log or actigraphy for 2 weeks can be utilized if the patient's personal account of a sleep-wake cycle is not clear or if there is doubt about the accuracy of the personal history.[2] Insufficient sleep syndrome may be more common in adolescence due to the higher sleep time needed, increased social pressure, and tendency toward a delayed sleep phase, which all lead to behavioral sleep restriction. Sleep deprivation in adolescents is common. The Youth Risk Behavior Survey found that 72.7% of students reported an average of <8 hours of sleep on school nights.[16] A variety of behaviors before bedtime are associated with worsening sleep metrics; hence, a discussion of the bedtime routine such as the use of electronic devices before bedtime is relevant history.[17]

Online Physical Examination

The telemedicine online physical examination for a patient complaining of hypersomnia should include an upper airway examination and a neurological examination. Please refer to Chapter 11 for details of the upper airway examination. EDS is a common symptom of OSA,[18] and clinical signs of upper airway crowding should be evaluated. In the telemedicine encounter, the clinician must observe the patient for manifestations of sleepiness such as lid lag, dozing during the interview, or consuming caffeine to counteract symptoms and help stay alert. The virtual examination may also help distinguish severe sleepiness from stupor due to neurological impairment or drugs.[19] If an underlying medical condition is suspected such as hypothyroidism, special attention on the skin for dryness, puffiness around the eyes, or a goiter on neck extension may be observed.[20]

Cerebral neurodegenerative disorders, such as Parkinson disease and dementia, are characterized by neuronal cell loss and abnormal accumulation of protein in cells in the brain.[10] If these degenerative areas of the brain affect wake-promoting areas such as the locus coeruleus, raphe nucleus, and hypocretin neurons, then hypersomnia may result.[10] Symptoms such as tremor, muscle rigidity, imbalance, and impaired cognition may be present. A focused virtual neurological examination may unveil important clinical signs suggesting an etiology for hypersomnia symptoms. A neurological examination may include these key testing points: mental status, cranial nerves, motor examination, sensory, gait, and coordination. Al Hussona et al.[21] created a procedure for virtual neurological testing. For the mental status portion, the provider can assess fluency of speech and appropriateness of affect and facial expressions. A question about recent history and stating the date, recent events, and counting backward may assess mental status. Cranial nerves and facial symmetry can be observed in a limited fashion. Lifting eyebrows, closing eyes tightly, showing teeth, and pursing lips may show any signs of asymmetry or weakness. Neck flexion, shrugging shoulders, and tongue protrusion and movement can complete the cranial nerve examination. For gross motor assessment, have the patient walk toward the camera and observe gait and arm swing. It may be possible to assess for pronator drift and for bradykinesia by asking patients to finger tap and open and close their fists. To evaluate coordination, ask patients to rapidly point from their nose to chin and heel to shin movements. A sensory examination may be difficult but may be achieved with patient participation. For example, the patient may be asked to hold an ice cube and check for equal sensation of the index finger or big toes on both sides of the body. Tremor can be evaluated by having patients attempt to grab an object (intention tremor) or by having patients hold their hands out in front of them at rest (resting tremor).

Management

Once the etiology of the hypersomnia is determined, treatment, often with medications, is initiated (Figures 12.1 and 12.2).[22] Depending on location, government regulations, and insurance requirements, some medications can be prescribed electronically.

Summary

In conclusion, the online history and physical examination in a telemedicine encounter should include questions that help guide the clinician to the differential diagnosis. The data collection will then help shape the next steps in diagnostic testing to confirm clinical suspicions. Patients presenting with hypersomnia may describe uncontrollable drowsiness, which may make driving

Recommended medications for narcolepsy in adult patients

Medication	Excessive daytime sleepiness	Cataplexy	Disease severity	Quality of life
Modafinil	●		●	●
Pitolisant	●	●	●	
Sodium Oxybate	●	●	●	
Solriamfetol	●		●	●
Armodafinil	●		●	
Dextroamphetamine	●	●		
Methylphenidate			●	

AASM clinical guideline
Strong recommendation: "We recommend..." almost all patients should receive the recommended course of action.
Conditional recommendation: "We suggest..." most patients should receive the suggested course of action.

Figure 12.1 Clinical practice guidelines for the pharmacological treatment of narcolepsy. *(Modified from Maski K, Trotti LM, Kotagal S, et al. Treatment of central disorders of hypersomnolence: an American Academy of Sleep Medicine clinical practice guideline.* J Clin Sleep Med. *2021;17[9]:1881-1893.)*

Recommended medications for idiopathic hypersomnia in adult patients

Medication	Excessive daytime sleepiness	Disease severity	Quality of life
Modafinil	●	●	
Clarithromycin	●	●	●
Methylphenidate		●	
Pitolisant	●		
Sodium Oxybate	●		

AASM clinical guideline
Strong recommendation: "We recommend..." almost all patients should receive the recommended course of action.
Conditional recommendation: "We suggest..." most patients should receive the suggested course of action.

Figure 12.2 Clinical practice guidelines for the pharmacological treatment of idiopathic hypersomnia. *(Modified from Maski K, Trotti LM, Kotagal S, et al. Treatment of central disorders of hypersomnolence: an American Academy of Sleep Medicine clinical practice guideline.* J Clin Sleep Med. *2021;17[9]:1881-1893.)*

or operating machinery unsafe, and ascertaining severity of symptoms is important for counseling and overall public safety. Various causes of hypersomnolence may range from central origin or underlying medical or psychiatric conditions to behavioral restrictions of sleep. A comprehensive sleep history along with medical history will also help navigate the focused virtual examination. The examination should be directed to some of the aforementioned etiologies and include an upper airway, head, and neck examination (as discussed in Chapter 10) and a neurological examination. The data obtained in a telemedicine encounter can be useful in management of patients with hypersomnia.

References

1. Ingravallo F, Vignatelli L, Pagotto U, et al. Protocols of a diagnostic study and a randomized controlled non-inferiority trial comparing televisits vs standard in-person outpatient visits for narcolepsy diagnosis and care: TElemedicine for NARcolepsy (TENAR). *BMC Neurol.* 2020;20(1):176. doi:10.1186/s12883-020-01762-9.
2. Pizza F, Vignatelli L, Oriolo C, et al. Multidisciplinary care of patients with narcolepsy during coronavirus disease 2019 pandemic in Italy via televisit: the TElemedicine for NARcolepsy feasibility study. *Sleep.* 2022;45(12):zsac228.
3. Uehli K, Mehta AJ, Miedinger D, et al. Sleep problems and work injuries: a systematic review and meta-analysis. *Sleep Med Rev.* 2014;18(1):61-73.
4. American Academy of Sleep Medicine. *ICSD-3, The International Classification of Sleep Disorders.* 3rd ed. Darien, IL: American Academy of Sleep Medicine; 2014.
5. Johns MW. A new method for measuring daytime sleepiness: the Epworth Sleepiness Scale. *Sleep.* 1991;14(6):540-545.
6. Vernet C, Leu-Semenescu S, Buzare MA, Arnulf I. Subjective symptoms in idiopathic hypersomnia: beyond excessive sleepiness. *J Sleep Res.* 2010;19(4):525-534.
7. Dauvilliers Y, Montplaisir J, Molinari N, et al. Age at onset of narcolepsy in two large populations of patients in France and Quebec. *Neurology.* 2001;57(11):2029-2033.
8. Won C, Mahmoudi M, Qin L, et al. The impact of gender on timeliness of narcolepsy diagnosis. *J Clin Sleep Med.* 2014;10(1):89-95.
9. Barateau L, Lopez R, Franchi JA, Dauvilliers Y. Hypersomnolence, hypersomnia, and mood disorders. *Curr Psychiatry Rep.* 2017;19(2):13.
10. Morgenthaler TI, Kapur VK, Brown T, et al. Practice parameters for the treatment of narcolepsy and other hypersomnias of central origin [published correction appears in Sleep. 2008;31(2):table of contents]. *Sleep.* 2007;30(12):1705-1711.
11. Singh J, Sharma BC, Puri V, Sachdeva S, Srivastava S. Sleep disturbances in patients of liver cirrhosis with minimal hepatic encephalopathy before and after lactulose therapy. *Metab Brain Dis.* 2017;32(2):595-605.
12. Malhotra RK. Neurodegenerative disorders and sleep. *Sleep Med Clin.* 2018;13(1):63-70.
13. Ding Q, Whittemore R, Redeker N. Excessive daytime sleepiness in stroke survivors: an integrative review. *Biol Res Nurs.* 2016;18(4):420-431.
14. Mbatchou Ngahane BH, Nganda MM, Dzudie A, et al. Prevalence and determinants of excessive daytime sleepiness in hypertensive patients: a cross-sectional study in Douala, Cameroon. *BMJ Open.* 2015;5(7):e008339.
15. Plante DT. Sleep propensity in psychiatric hypersomnolence: a systematic review and meta-analysis of multiple sleep latency test findings. *Sleep Med Rev.* 2017;31:48-57.
16. Wheaton AG, Jones SE, Cooper AC, Croft JB. Short sleep duration among middle school and high school students—United States, 2015. *MMWR Morb Mortal Wkly Rep.* 2018;67(3):85-90.
17. Levenson JC, Shensa A, Sidani JE, Colditz JB, Primack BA. Social media use before bed and sleep disturbance among young adults in the United States: a nationally representative study. *Sleep.* 2017;40(9):zsx113.
18. He K, Kapur VK. Sleep-disordered breathing and excessive daytime sleepiness. *Sleep Med Clin.* 2017;12(3):369-382.
19. Kryger M, Roth T, Dement B. *Principles and Practice of Sleep Medicine.* 6th ed. Philadelphia: Elsevier; 2017.
20. McDermott MT. Hypothyroidism. *Ann Intern Med.* 2020;173(1):ITC1-ITC16.
21. Al Hussona M, Maher M, Chan D, et al. The virtual neurologic exam: instructional videos and guidance for the COVID-19 era. *Can J Neurol Sci.* 2020;47(5):598-603.
22. Maski K, Trotti LM, Kotagal S, et al. Treatment of central disorders of hypersomnolence: an American Academy of Sleep Medicine clinical practice guideline. *J Clin Sleep Med.* 2021;17(9):1881-1893.

CHAPTER **13**

Circadian Rhythm Sleep-Wake Disorders

Vivian Asare

Introduction

Most circadian rhythm sleep-wake disorders (CRSWDs) occur when there is recurrent disturbance of the alignment between a patient's internal circadian rhythm and timing requirements of work, social activities, and school. Some of the disorders are *intrinsic* (related to the patient's underlying circadian rhythm), while others are *extrinsic* (related to external factors such as lifestyle, work schedules, or travel). Patients will often present with symptoms of hypersomnolence or insomnia as a result of the misalignment. An online history should include the patient's pattern of sleep-wake cycle on both weekdays and on weekends (or when the patient does not have environmental time constraints affecting their sleep schedule). Sleep logs and actigraphy can help provide essential information in accurately classifying the type of CRSWD. Utilizing questionnaires such as the Horne-Ostberg Morningness-Eveningness Questionnaire (MEQ)[1] and the Munich Chronotype Questionnaire (MCTQ),[2] which evaluate circadian preference (also known as *chronotype*), may also aid in diagnosis and treatment. The MEQ is the most common questionnaire used to assess chronotype; it is a 19-item self-assessment that evaluates personal preference of the timing of sleep and other activities. In this chapter, we will discuss each type of CRSWD and the approach to the online history based on presenting symptoms in a telemedicine encounter.

DELAYED SLEEP-WAKE PHASE DISORDER

In delayed sleep-wake phase disorder (DSWPD), there is a significant delay between the phase of the major sleep episode and the desired or required sleep-wake cycle. This discrepancy leads to complaints of difficulty falling asleep and awakening at the required times.[3] When patients are allowed to set their own schedule, these symptoms resolve, and the patient maintains a stable delayed 24-hour cycle. Individuals with DSWPD naturally do not fall asleep until the early morning hours and wake up in the late morning or early afternoon. During their preferred sleep schedules, sleep duration and quality are generally normal.[4] The online clinical sleep interview should include the patient's report on their sleep-wake cycle on both workdays and free days. Patients may describe sleep-onset insomnia, however, asking specifically during the encounter about sleep latency when they are able to go to sleep at their preferred delayed time will reveal that their latency is no longer increased.[5] Sleep logs and actigraphy should be maintained for at least 7 consecutive days, and preferably for 14 days. These logs will show delayed sleep onset and offset, usually by more than 2 hours past socially acceptable times.[3] Daytime sleepiness on awakening at the required versus the preferred time may be reported, and questions to screen for other sleep disorders that may cause daytime sleepiness, such as sleep-disordered breathing, psychiatric disorders, and medical disorders, should be included in the history. Insomnia may co-occur with DSWPD[6] along with other psychiatric disorders such as bipolar disorder[7] and severe obsessive-compulsive disorder.[8]

121

ADVANCED SLEEP-WAKE PHASE DISORDER

In advanced sleep-wake phase disorder (ASWPD), there is a sleep pattern scheduled several hours earlier than is usual or desired. There is no standard for how much earlier a sleep schedule must be in order to qualify as pathological.[4] Patients may describe a history of being unable to stay awake until their desired or required bedtime and being unable to stay asleep until their desired wake time. The clinician should also evaluate for other potential causes of sleep maintenance insomnia. Advanced age tends to be a risk factor, with older age being highly associated with increased morningness. It is important to evaluate older adults for other potential causes for maintenance insomnia and evening sleepiness, such as sleep-disordered breathing and movement disorders, because these also have a higher incidence in older adults.[9]

SHIFT WORK DISORDER

Shift work refers to non-standard work schedules, including night work, early morning work, and rotating schedules. Shift work disorder results when patients develop sleep disturbance and daytime dysfunction due to their non-conventional work schedule. Patients may describe in the clinical history that they have difficulty falling asleep after a night shift, or they may have impairment in waking alertness and performance. Total sleep time is often curtailed by about 1 to 4 hours, and sleep quality is described as poor.[3] The clinical interview for shift workers should include a discussion about their work history, detailed sleep history, and impairments during wakefulness. A comprehensive work history should include occupation, work schedule, number of shifts per week, and how long they have been on the shift schedule. Sleep patterns should be assessed separately for both on-shift and off-shift periods. About 20% of U.S. workers are involved in shift work, and about 10% of the U.S. workforce experience sleep disturbance and sleepiness severe enough to meet the criteria for shift work disorder.[10] An epidemiological study found that workers on a rotating shift show increased odds of obesity (odds ratio, 1.57; 95% confidence interval [CI], 1.12–2.21), with a significant trend of increasing odds with longer duration of shift work.[11] These patients are at high risk for sleep-disordered breathing, and an assessment for this should be included in the clinical interview. Individuals have varying degrees of adaptability to shift work. Social pressures before and after a work shift can affect sleep duration in shift workers and cause short sleep time. Discussing a patient's routine before and after a shift is helpful to understand ways to improve sleep duration.

JET LAG DISORDER

Patients with jet lag disorder will provide a history of recent trans-meridian travel of at least two time zones, and they will complain of insomnia or daytime sleepiness and a reduction of sleep time. Symptoms such as malaise, fatigue, or somatic complaints will occur within 1 to 2 days after travel. The severity and duration are dependent on the number of time zones traveled and is temporary.[3] Eastward travel causes difficulty with sleep onset and daytime sleepiness because of a misalignment between internal circadian time and the travelers' biological clock. Westward travel leads to sleepiness in the evening and early morning awakenings. Symptoms are temporary, and it is estimated that it takes 1 day per time zone for circadian rhythm recovery.[12]

IRREGULAR SLEEP-WAKE RHYTHM DISORDER

Patients with irregular sleep-wake rhythm disorder (ISWRD) will give a history of chronic or recurrent periods of irregular sleep and wake episodes throughout a 24-hour cycle. Patients will complain of insomnia during sleep periods and daytime sleepiness during wake periods. A sleep log or actigraphy monitored for at least 7 days will reveal no major sleep period and at least three irregular sleep bouts in a 24-hour period. This irregularity is not explained by any other current sleep, medical, neurological, or psychiatric disorder.[3] ISWRD is most commonly found in older adults with neurodegenerative disorders or psychiatric disorders or in children with neurodevelopmental delay.[13] In the reported history, patients may state difficulty synchronizing sleep to socially normal times, and the sleep fragmentation will include frequent napping throughout the day, with the longest sleep periods lasting less than 4 hours.[14] The longest sleep times usually are from 2:00 AM to 6:00 AM. Total sleep time usually is within the normal range for age within a 24-hour period, but patients will describe an inability to consolidate sleep into a single 6- to 8-hour period.[15] As a result, this disorder is characterized by a lack of a clearly defined circadian sleep and wake cycle.[13] In the clinical interview, patients typically describe sleep maintenance insomnia,[4] and it is usually the most difficult symptom for caregivers to experience. Actigraphy along with a sleep diary over a 7- to 14-day period has the most utility in accurately diagnosing this disorder.[15] An actigraph shows a disturbed low-amplitude circadian rhythm with a loss of normal diurnal sleep-wake patterns. An essential part of the history is distinguishing the irregular sleep-wake pattern from other sleep disorders associated with poor sleep hygiene or a voluntary maintenance of an irregular schedule, such as shift work.[15]

NON-24-HOUR SLEEP WAKE RHYTHM DISORDER (N24SWRD)

In the clinical online history, patients will describe insomnia, excessive daytime sleepiness, or both. These symptoms will alternate with asymptomatic periods due to misalignment between the 24-hour light-dark cycle and the non-entrained endogenous circadian rhythm of sleep-wake propensity.[3] There will be a pattern of progressive delay of sleep-wake times as the circadian period is usually longer than 24 hours.[3] Episodes of sleep disturbance will typically start with progressive increase in sleep latency and delay in sleep onset. The propensity rhythm then shifts into the daytime; patients will start reporting difficulty falling asleep at night and staying awake during the day. As the sleep-wake propensity continues to drift, patients will then report late afternoon and evening sleepiness with frequent napping as well as early sleep onset and shortened sleep latency. N24SWRD has been described in up to 63% of blind individuals who lack light perception, thought to be due to the lack of photic input to the suprachiasmatic nucleus[16]; however, this disorder also can be seen in sighted individuals. In the largest case series of sighted individuals, 57 people were described with N24SWRD,[17] 72% were male, and the majority began to exhibit symptoms in their teens or 20s. Similar to patients with DSWPD, there seems to be a high comorbidity of psychiatric disorders in sighted patients with N24SWRD. In this case series, 28% of patients had a pre-morbid psychiatric disorder prior to developing N24SWD, and 25% developed symptoms of major depression after the onset of N24SWRD.[17] A sighted patient with suspected N24SWRD may report first having a delayed sleep phase–type onset of sleep between the hours of 3:00 AM to 6:00 AM and then gradually progressing to a non-24-hour sleep-wake cycle.[18] This makes monitoring sleep logs and actigraphy for greater than 14 days essential.

Online Physical Examination

The online physical examination for a patient suspected of having a circadian rhythm disorder should include an upper airway examination (refer to Chapter 11 for details on the telemedicine upper airway examination), neurological examination (refer to Chapter 12 for details on the telemedicine neurological examination), and a viewing of the patient's bedroom environment. CRSWDs can cause insomnia and daytime sleepiness symptoms, and it is important to evaluate for other possible etiologies, such as sleep-disordered breathing, movement disorders of sleep, neurological disorders, or environmental behavioral causes. Shift workers are more likely to be obese,[11] placing them at risk for sleep-disordered breathing. Night shift workers may have bedroom environments that are not conducive to sleeping during the day, and a view of the bedroom environment may provide some insight into reported insomnia issues. Individuals with DSWPD, ISWRD, and N24SWRD may not be exposed to enough sunlight or other zeitgebers, which may perpetuate irregular sleep-wake patterns.[3] In the case of DSWPD, not enough sunlight exposure in the morning or too much light in the evening may further delay their sleep.[3] A dark room during the clinical interview may provide clues to this finding. Patients with ISWRD are most commonly older adults with neurodegenerative disorders,[13] and a focused neurological examination is recommended.

Tools to Monitor Circadian Rhythms

Sleep diaries and actigraphs[19] are the most widely used instruments that can be used by patients in the home setting. Consumer wearables can be used.[20,21] Even more sophisticated home monitoring systems have been employed.[22]

Management Guidelines

Management guidelines have been published for intrinsic[23] and extrinsic[24] circadian sleep-wake disorders.

Conclusion

In this chapter, we discussed the main types of CRSWDs. In a telemedicine interview, patients may only complain of significant insomnia or daytime sleepiness, and it will be the clinicians' history taking and thorough questioning that will help distinguish these disorders from other sleep disorders such as primary insomnia or a disorder of hypersomnolence. A 7- to 14-day sleep history and/or actigraphy is an essential part of understanding the sleep pattern of patients on both weekdays and weekends and how it may change over time. The circadian preference versus social, school, travel, and work requirements may cause a misalignment and subsequent disturbance in the sleep-wake cycle. Utilizing questionnaires such as the MEQ[1] may also aid in diagnosis and treatment.

References

1. Horne JA, Ostberg O. A self-assessment questionnaire to determine morningness-eveningness in human circadian rhythms. *Int J Chronobiol.* 1976;4(2):97-110.
2. Roenneberg T, Wirz-Justice A, Merrow M. Life between clocks: daily temporal patterns of human chronotypes. *J Biol Rhythms.* 2003;18(1):80-90.
3. American Academy of Sleep Medicine. *ICSD-3, The International Classification of Sleep Disorders.* 3rd ed. Darien, IL: American Academy of Sleep Medicine; 2014.
4. Auger RR, Burgess HJ, Emens JS, et al. Clinical practice guideline for the treatment of intrinsic circadian rhythm sleep-wake disorders: advanced sleep-wake phase disorder (ASWPD), delayed sleep-wake phase disorder (DSWPD), non-24-hour sleep-wake rhythm disorder (N24SWD), and irregular sleep-wake rhythm disorder (ISWRD). An update for 2015. *J Clin Sleep Med.* 2015;11(10):1199-1236.
5. Culnan E, McCullough LM, Wyatt JK. Circadian rhythm sleep-wake phase disorders. *Neurol Clin.* 2019;37(3):527-543.
6. Sivertsen B, Pallesen S, Stormark KM, et al. Delayed sleep phase syndrome in adolescents: prevalence and correlates in a large population based study. *BMC Public Health.* 2013;13:1163.
7. Robillard R, Naismith S L, Rogers NL, et al. Delayed sleep phase in young people with unipolar or bipolar affective disorders. *J Affect Disord.* 2013;145(2):260-263.

8. Turner J, Drummond LM, Mukhopadhyay S, et al. A prospective study of delayed sleep phase syndrome in patients with severe resistant obsessive-compulsive disorder. *World Psychiatry*. 2007;6(2):108-111.
9. Yaremchuk K. Sleep disorders in the elderly. *Clin Geriatr Med*. 2018;34(2):205-216.
10. Cheng P, Drake C. Shift work disorder. *Neurol Clin*. 2019;37(3):563-577.
11. Grundy A, Cotterchio M, Kirsh VA, et al. Rotating shift work associated with obesity in men from northeastern Ontario. Association entre le travail par quarts et l'obésité chez les hommes dans le nord-est de l'Ontario. *Health Promot Chronic Dis Prev Can*. 2017;37(8):238-247.
12. Reid KJ, Abbott SM. Jet lag and shift work disorder. *Sleep Med Clin*. 2015;10(4):523-535.
13. Oyegbile T, Videnovic A. Irregular sleep-wake rhythm disorder. *Neurol Clin*. 2019;37(3):553-561.
14. Pavlova M. Circadian rhythm sleep-wake disorders. *Continuum. (Minneap Minn)*. 2017;23(4):1051-1063.
15. Abbott SM, Zee PC. Irregular sleep-wake rhythm disorder. *Sleep Med Clin*. 2015;10(4):517-522.
16. Flynn-Evans EE, Tabandeh H, Skene DJ, et al. Circadian rhythm disorders and melatonin production in 127 blind women with and without light perception. *J Biol Rhythms*. 2014;29(3):215-224.
17. Hayakawa T, Uchiyama M, Kamei Y, et al. Clinical analyses of sighted patients with non-24-hour sleep-wake syndrome: a study of 57 consecutively diagnosed cases. *Sleep*. 2005;28(8):945-952.
18. Malkani RG, Abbott SM, Reid KJ, et al. Diagnostic and treatment challenges of sighted non-24-hour sleep-wake disorder. *J Clin Sleep Med*. 2018;14(4):603-613.
19. Smith MT, McCrae CS, Cheung J, et al. Use of actigraphy for the evaluation of sleep disorders and circadian rhythm sleep-wake disorders. An American Academy of Sleep Medicine Clinical Practice Guideline. *J Clin Sleep Med*. 2018;14(7):1231-1237.
20. Tahara Y, Shinto T, Inoue K, et al. Changes in sleep phase and body weight of mobile health app users during COVID-19 mild lockdown in Japan. *Int J Obes (Lond)*. 2021;45(10):2277-2280.
21. Schutte-Rodin S, Deak MC, Khosla S, et al. Evaluating consumer and clinical sleep technologies: an American Academy of Sleep Medicine update. *J Clin Sleep Med*. 2021;17(11):2275-2282.
22. Zhang Y, Cordina-Duverger E, Komarzynski S, et al. Digital circadian and sleep health in individual hospital shift workers: a cross sectional telemonitoring study. *EBioMedicine*. 2022;81:104121.
23. Auger RR, Burgess HJ, Emens JS, Deriy LV, Thomas SM, Sharkey KM. Clinical practice guideline for the treatment of intrinsic circadian rhythm sleep-wake disorders. Advanced sleep-wake phase disorder (AS-WPD), delayed sleep-wake phase disorder (DSWPD), non-24-hour sleep-wake rhythm disorder (N24SWD), and irregular sleep-wake rhythm disorder (ISWRD). An update for 2015: an American Academy of Sleep Medicine Clinical Practice Guideline. *J Clin Sleep Med*. 2015;11(10):1199-1236.
24. Morgenthaler TI, Lee-Chiong T, Alessi C, et al. Practice parameters for the clinical evaluation and treatment of circadian rhythm sleep disorders. An American Academy of Sleep Medicine report [published correction appears in Sleep. 2008;31(7):table of contents]. *Sleep*. 2007;30(11):1445-1459.

CHAPTER 14

Sleep-Related Movement Disorders

Vivian Asare

Online History
RESTLESS LEGS SYNDROME

Restless legs syndrome (RLS), also known as *Willis-Ekbom disease*, is a common sensorimotor disorder that affects the legs, and in some cases the upper extremities. RLS can significantly disrupt sleep initiation and maintenance and impair daytime function and overall quality of life.[1] The prevalence of RLS is between 3% and 29% of the general population in Western countries.[2] About 2.7% of individuals report moderately disruptive symptoms that would warrant treatment, and of this group, 55.5% report daytime dysfunction due to symptoms.[3] During an online history, patients may describe having an overwhelming urge to move the legs (or other body parts) and that these symptoms worsen during rest and in the evening. Repositioning or getting up to move often alleviates the urge. RLS is thought to be a central nervous system disorder related to brain iron insufficiency and dopaminergic dysfunction.[4] Assessing the time of onset, location, exacerbating factors, consumption of caffeine or alcohol, and the medication list evaluation are important parts of the online history. Patients may commonly use the following descriptors: "twitchy," "need to stretch," "urge to move," and "legs want to move on their own."[5] About one-half of patients with RLS may describe the sensation as painful.[5] Common conditions that may mimic RLS in a patient history are leg cramps, habitual leg tapping, peripheral neuropathy, leg edema, arthritis, and myalgias.

The three conditions that are most commonly associated with RLS are pregnancy, iron deficiency, and end-stage renal disease. Patients with these underlying conditions are at high risk, and suspicion should be high during the clinical interview. RLS is present in 25% to 35% of patients with iron deficiency anemia, and in pregnancy, the severity and prevalence of RLS increases with each passing trimester and tends to resolve after delivery.[6] Epidemiological studies have also shown an association between RLS and mood disorders, such as anxiety, depression, and panic disorder; this is independent of antidepressant use.[7] Antidepressants can precipitate or worsen RLS in 9% of patients, and mirtazapine is most commonly associated with this effect (28%).[8] A comprehensive medical history and medication list will provide important information regarding risk factors and modifiable exogenous precipitants. RLS severity can be assessed using the Restless Legs Syndrome Rating Scale, which the patient fills in.

Idiopathic Hypersomnia Severity Scale

Restless Legs Syndrome Rating Scale

Your name/code number: _____ Today's Date: _____
                              last, first   month/day/year

Carefully read each question and all answers
What day was 7 days ago?
Think about your RLS during that day and **the next 7 days** up to today <u>not</u> just the most recent or RLS worse days.
Report the **usual (not most or least severe)** effects of only RLS during the past 7 days regardless of any medications changes during that time
Report **effects of only RLS** <u>not</u> other life or health problems in this past week

Self-Completed International Restless Legs Syndrome Study Group Severity Rating Scale (sIRLS)

In the past week...
 (1) <u>Overall</u>, how would you rate the <u>RLS discomfort in your legs or arms</u>?
     4☐ Very severe
     3☐ Severe
     2☐ Moderate
     1☐ Mild
     0☐ None

In the past week...
 (2) <u>Overall</u>, how would you rate the <u>need to move</u> around because of your RLS symptoms?
     4☐ Very severe
     3☐ Severe
     2☐ Moderate
     1☐ Mild
     0☐ None

In the past week...
 (3) <u>Overall</u>, how much <u>relief</u> from your RLS arm or leg discomfort did you get from moving around?
     4☐ No relief
     3☐ Mild relief
     2☐ Moderate relief
     1☐ Either complete or almost complete relief
     0☐ No RLS symptoms to be relieved

In the past week...

(4) How severe was your <u>sleep disturbance</u> due to your RLS symptoms?

        4☐ Very severe
        3☐ Severe
        2☐ Moderate
        1☐ Mild
        0☐ None

In the past week...

(5) How severe was your <u>tiredness</u> or <u>sleepiness</u> <u>during the day</u> due to your RLS symptoms?

        4☐ Very severe
        3☐ Severe
        2☐ Moderate
        1☐ Mild
        0☐ None

In the past week...

(6) How severe was <u>your RLS on the whole</u>?

        4☐ Very severe
        3☐ Severe
        2☐ Moderate
        1☐ Mild
        0☐ None

In the past week...

(7) How <u>often</u> did you get RLS symptoms?

        4☐ Very often (This means 6–7 days per week)
        3☐ Often (This means 4–5 days per week)
        2☐ Sometimes (This means 2–3 days per week)
        1☐ Occasionally (This means 1 day a week)
        0☐ Never

In the past week...

(8) When you had RLS symptoms, how severe were they on average?

        4☐ Very severe (This means 8 hours or more per 24-hour day)
        3☐ Severe (This means 3–8 hours per 24-hour day)
        2☐ Moderate (This means 1–3 hours per 24-hour day)
        1☐ Mild (This means less than 1 hour per 24-hour day)
        0☐ None

Continued

In the past week...

(9) <u>Overall</u>, how severe was the impact of your RLS symptoms on your ability to carry out your <u>daily activities</u>, for example having a satisfactory family, home, social, school or work life?

    4☐ Very severe
    3☐ Severe
    2☐ Moderate
    1☐ Mild
    0☐ None

In the past week...

(10) How severe was your <u>mood disturbance</u> due to your RLS symptoms – for example being angry, depressed, sad, anxious or irritable?

    4☐ Very severe
    3☐ Severe
    2☐ Moderate
    1☐ Mild
    0☐ None

Supplemental question:

(11) How do your usual RLS symptoms over a year compare to RLS symptoms for the last 7 days – which you reported above (circle the words)

Usual symptoms are worse

    1. Extremely worse
    2. Much worse
    3. Somewhat worse
    4. About the same

Usual symptoms are better

    5. Somewhat better
    6. Much better
    7. Extremely better

Comments:

PERIODIC LIMB MOVEMENT DISORDER

Periodic limb movement disorder (PLMD) is characterized by highly stereotyped limb movements occurring during sleep and is associated with sleep disturbance or daytime dysfunction. These symptoms cannot be attributed to another primary sleep disorder such as RLS, obstructive sleep apnea (OSA), narcolepsy, or REM behavior disorder.[5] Periodic limb movements of sleep (PLMS) most commonly occur in the lower extremities and involve extension of the big toe and flexion of the ankle, knee, and sometimes the hip. In the patient history, a bed partner may complain of sleep disturbance from the nocturnal movements. These movements can be associated with an autonomic response, arousals, sleep fragmentation, and subsequent daytime sleepiness.[9] The presence of clinical symptoms is what differentiates PLMD from isolated PLMS. PLMS are common in RLS, occurring in up to 80% to 90% of RLS patients, though patients with PLMS may not commonly have RLS.[10] A positive family history of RLS increases the risk for PLMD and PLMs, so obtaining a thorough family history is an important part of the clinical interview. The gene variants *BTBD9* and *MEIS1*, found in genome studies of RLS, have also been found to influence the expression of PLMS.[11] In a recent cohort study, patients with PLMS were more likely to be on medications such as hypnotics, beta blockers, antidepressants, antihistamines, and neuroleptic agents. A complete medication list is essential in evaluating various risk factors and possible causes for PLMS and PLMD.[11] In this sleep cohort study, the prevalence of PLMS in the general population was found to be 28.6%; these patients were older, with a higher percentage of males and post-menopausal females and a higher body mass index (BMI). A higher percentage of subjects had RLS, diabetes, and hypertension, with a lower mean glomerular filtration rate.[11] A comprehensive clinical online history in evaluating a patient suspected of having PLMD should involve an assessment for an underlying primary sleep disorder, family history, current medication use, and medical history. The clinical significance beyond sleep disturbance in some individuals with PLMS is unknown, and treatment is often dictated by clinical symptoms.

PROPRIOSPINAL MYOCLONUS AT SLEEP ONSET

Propriospinal myoclonus (PSM) at sleep onset is characterized by sudden myoclonic jerks that occur during the transition from wakefulness to sleep. The sudden movement occurs mainly in the abdomen, trunk, and neck. They first occur as flexion in the abdomen and trunk and then propagate to the proximal muscles of the limbs and neck. These jerking movements disrupt sleep onset, and patients will complain of severe sleep onset insomnia.[5] These movements can sometimes be precipitated by external stimuli, but they usually occur spontaneously and disappear with mental activation and the transition to stable sleep. PSM should be distinguished from hypnic jerks, which are common and physiological with no clear pattern of propriospinal propagation.[12] The prevalence is higher in males and thought to be quite rare. It starts in adulthood, and it is unremitting and usually chronic. Patients may describe a fear of falling asleep that is associated with depression and anxiety. If the movement is severe enough, it could cause injury to the patient or bed partner.[5]

SLEEP-RELATED BRUXISM

The International Classification of Sleep Disorders describes sleep-related bruxism as the presence of regular or frequent tooth-grinding sounds occurring during sleep and the presence of either abnormal tooth wear or transient morning jaw muscle pain or fatigue, or temporal headache or jaw locking consistent with a history of tooth grinding. Patients may complain of tooth pain, jaw pain, jaw locking, or temporal headaches. Dentists may often refer patients after noticing on evaluation abnormal tooth wear and damage from frequent grinding. A bed partner may complain of an unpleasant noise made during sleep, and if severe, a patient may have associated sleep disruption from symptoms.[5] Complaints of abnormal tooth and jaw sensations and headaches localized to the temporal area are frequently reported. There is a correlation between stress and anxiety and sleep-related bruxism. Secondary sleep-related bruxism is bruxism caused by an underlying condition such as medication use, recreational drug use, or a medical disorder such as RBD or Parkinson disease. Caffeine and nicotine use prior to bedtime can increase the frequency of bruxism as a result of arousals. Bruxism can also be familial; 20% to 50% of patients with sleep-related bruxism report that at least one family member also suffers from similar symptoms.[13]

Online Physical Examination

The telemedicine online physical examination for a patient suspected of a sleep-related movement disorder should include an upper airway examination and neurological examination. Please refer to Chapter 11 for details of the upper airway examination and Chapter 12 for details of the neurological examination.

With the evaluation of RLS and PLMD, other possible etiologies of lower leg symptoms such as lower extremity edema, venous insufficiency, arthritis, and peripheral neuropathy should be assessed.[5] Observe leg skin turgor, assess for swelling or asymmetry, and ask the patient to palpate shins and ankles for pitting edema. Look for swollen knee joints and ask the patient about tenderness to palpation of the joints or whether there is audible crepitus with range of motion. A comprehensive neurological examination is indicated because RLS and PLMS can be associated with other neurological diseases, such as neuropathy, multiple sclerosis, or Parkinson disease.[14] Although telemedicine limits a comprehensive neurological examination, some important observations may be obtained such as the presence of resting or intentional tremors, abnormal gait, dysarthria, and cognitive assessments. Telemedicine management of patients with movement disorders proved feasible during the coronavirus disease 2019 (COVID-19) pandemic.[15]

Sleep-related movement disorders may also be associated with sleep-disordered breathing, such as OSA. A thorough upper airway examination may reveal airway crowding or other findings that may increase suspicion for an underlying primary sleep disorder (see Chapter 11).

Online physical examination for suspected bruxism should involve an oral examination of dentition. Have the patient show all teeth and assess for chipped or broken teeth, which may suggest repetitive friction from tooth grinding. Tooth surface loss may also be observed. Tenderness in the masseter muscles and temporalis muscle regions may be present, and a clinician can ask the patient to palpate this area and report whether tenderness is elicited. Hypertrophy of the masseter and temporal muscles may also be present.[16]

MANAGEMENT

Guidelines are available for the management of movement disorders (RLS[17] and RBD[18]) affecting sleep. Because some of the treatments of movement disorders may require scheduled medication, the prescriber will be bound by local regulations for using such compounds.

In conclusion, sleep-related movement disorders are characterized by simple movements during sleep causing sleep maintenance or onset disturbance. Patients may complain of insomnia or associated daytime sleepiness. During a telemedicine encounter, a comprehensive history involving the timing, onset, exacerbating factors, location, frequency, and severity of symptoms will assist in finding the correct diagnosis along with polysomnographic evidence in some cases. The clinical interview should also include medication use, family history, and medical history as certain medications can exacerbate movements, some familial patterns of occurrence exist, and certain medical disorders confer a higher risk for developing movement disorders. The online physical examination, although limited, may yield some helpful upper airway and neurological examination findings.

References

1. Trotti LM. Restless legs syndrome and sleep-related movement disorders. *Continuum (Minneap Minn)*. 2017;23(4, Sleep Neurology):1005-1016.
2. Innes KE, Selfe TK, Agarwal P. Prevalence of restless legs syndrome in North American and Western European populations: a systematic review. *Sleep Med*. 2011;12(7):623-634.
3. Allen RP, Walters AS, Montplaisir J, et al. Restless legs syndrome prevalence and impact: REST general population study. *Arch Intern Med*. 2005;165(11):1286-1292.
4. Earley CJ, Connor J, Garcia-Borreguero D, et al. Altered brain iron homeostasis and dopaminergic function in restless legs syndrome (Willis-Ekbom disease). *Sleep Med*. 2014;15(11):1288-1301.
5. American Academy of Sleep Medicine. *ICSD-3, The International Classification of Sleep Disorders*. 3rd ed. TR. Darien, IL: American Academy of Sleep Medicine; 2023.

6. Trenkwalder C, Allen R, Högl B, et al. Restless legs syndrome associated with major diseases: a systematic review and new concept. *Neurology.* 2016;86(14):1336-1343.
7. Becker PM, Sharon D. Mood disorders in restless legs syndrome (Willis-Ekbom disease). *J Clin Psychiatry.* 2014;75(7):e679-e694.
8. Rottach KG, Schaner BM, Kirch MH, et al. Restless legs syndrome as side effect of second generation antidepressants. *J Psychiatr Res.* 2008;43(1):70-75.
9. Aurora RN, Kristo DA, Bista SR, et al. Update to the AASM clinical practice guideline: "The treatment of restless legs syndrome and periodic limb movement disorder in adults—an update for 2012: practice parameters with an evidence-based systematic review and meta-analyses." *Sleep.* 2012;35(8):1037.
10. Walters AS, Rye DB. Review of the relationship of restless legs syndrome and periodic limb movements in sleep to hypertension, heart disease, and stroke. *Sleep.* 2009;32(5):589-597. In press.
11. Haba-Rubio J, Marti-Soler H, Marques-Vidal P, et al. Prevalence and determinants of periodic limb movements in the general population. *Ann Neurol.* 2016;79(3):464-474.
12. Stefani A, Högl B. Diagnostic criteria, differential diagnosis, and treatment of minor motor activity and less well-known movement disorders of sleep. *Curr Treat Options Neurol.* 2019;21(1):1.
13. Lobbezoo F, Ahlberg J, Raphael KG, et al. International consensus on the assessment of bruxism: report of a work in progress. *J Oral Rehabil.* 2018;45(11):837-844.
14. Kryger M, Roth T, Dement B. *Principles and Practice of Sleep Medicine.* 7th ed. Philadelphia: Elsevier; 2022.
15. Lima DP, Gomes VC, Viana Júnior AB, et al. Telehealth for Parkinson disease patients during the COVID-19 pandemic: the TeleParkinson study. Telesaúde para pacientes com doença de Parkinson durante a pandemia de COVID-19: o estudo TeleParkinson. *Arq Neuropsiquiatr.* 2022;80(10):1026-1035.
16. Beddis H, Pemberton M, Davies S. Sleep bruxism: an overview for clinicians. *Br Dent J.* 2018;225(6):497-501.
17. Anguelova GV, Vlak MHM, Kurvers AGY, Rijsman RM. Pharmacologic and nonpharmacologic treatment of restless legs syndrome. *Sleep Med Clin.* 2020;15(2):277-288.
18. Howell M, Avidan AY, Foldvary-Schaefer N, et al. Management of REM sleep behavior disorder: an American Academy of Sleep Medicine clinical practice guideline. *J Clin Sleep Med.* 2023;19(4):759-768.

CHAPTER 15

Telehealth CBT-I

Lynelle Schneeberg　■　Susan Rubman

Introduction

The term *insomnia* is used both clinically and colloquially to describe difficulty with sleep, generally in reference to insufficient, disrupted, or non-restorative sleep. The American Academy of Sleep Medicine and Sleep Research Society 2015 Consensus Statement indicates that, for adults, 7 to 9 hours of sleep per night on a regular basis is recommended to promote optimal health.[1] Inherent in this statement is the recognition that there is some natural variability in normal human sleep, both within individuals on a nightly basis and also among individuals in general. Sleep also has natural variability under certain physical or psychosocial events or circumstances. It is common, even predictable, to experience an occasional night of sleeplessness or time-limited sleep difficulties associated with these events. Sleep may be considered problematic, or of clinical significance, however, when it persistently deviates from the recommended guidelines or results in impairment in an individual's daytime functioning.

The *International Classification of Sleep Disorders*, third edition, and the *Diagnostic and Statistical Manual of Mental Disorders*, fifth edition, delineate the current classification and diagnostic systems for insomnia.[2,3] Both are generally aligned in the definitions and criteria for insomnia.

Diagnostic criteria include the following:

- Complaint of difficulty initiating sleep, difficulty maintaining sleep, and/or early morning awakenings with an inability to return to sleep
- Daytime consequences, distress, or impairment associated with the sleep difficulties
- Sleep disturbance occurs at least three times per week
- Duration of at least 3 months
- Sleep difficulty occurs despite adequate opportunity for sleep
- Symptoms are not better explained by another disorder and are not attributable to a substance

Insomnia *symptoms* occur in as much as 33% to 50% of the adult population, and rates can vary by demographic factors including age, gender, socioeconomic status, and health status.[3,4] Overall prevalence estimates of chronic insomnia *disorder* are lower, with an estimated prevalence of 6% to 10%.[3]

Cognitive behavioral therapy for insomnia (CBT-I) is a multicomponent therapy that typically includes stimulus control training, sleep restriction, cognitive therapy aimed at addressing misconceptions and inaccurate beliefs about sleep, sleep education, and sleep hygiene guidelines.[5] It may also contain components of relaxation training. It has been delivered successfully for individuals and in group settings. CBT-I is a short-term therapy and is generally conducted over a limited number of visits.

CBT-I is efficacious and has been found to yield improvement in the majority of patients, with gains well maintained over time.[6,7] CBT-I has been studied in a variety of populations including patients with breast cancer, obstructive sleep apnea, chronic pain, and psychiatric populations as well as in older adults.[6,8,9] CBT-I is recommended as the standard or first-line treatment by multiple professional bodies including the American College of Physicians, the British Association for

Psychopharmacology, The American Academy of Sleep Medicine, and the European Sleep Research Society.[10-14]

Limitations of CBT-I have included the relative scarcity of trained providers and distance required to travel to available providers, which can leave patients without access to effective treatment. Strategies to increase treatment availability have included the exploration of alternative types of treatment delivery, most notably via electronic media. These strategies have included both synchronous and asynchronous treatments.[15,16] In addition, strategies have included varying levels of provider contact, ranging from Internet-based manualized self-study treatment with automated feedback and application-based treatments to greater degrees of provider intervention with telephone-based therapy and video-based therapy.[17-22] Meta-analyses reveal that the use of Internet-delivered CBT-I is supported, and specifically that greater clinician involvement produces greater patient improvement.[23]

More recently and with the increased availability of webcams and smart technology video devices, CBT-I has been delivered via audiovisual telehealth services in the same manner and with the same content as treatment provided in a clinic setting. The remainder of the chapter will use the term *telehealth CBT-I* to refer to treatment that is essentially identical to face-to-face treatment but delivered via audiovisual telehealth services. Beginning with feasibility studies, advancing to randomized controlled trials and subsequent evaluation through meta-analyses, telehealth CBT-I has been shown to be an effective method of insomnia treatment, yielding statistically and clinically significant differences in standardized measures of sleep as well as improvements in sleep diary measures.[23-27]

Also helping to establish telehealth CBT-I as a credible and valuable treatment modality, Arnedt and colleagues compared telehealth CBT-I to face-to-face CBT-I in a randomized control non-inferiority trial.[28] Treatment acceptability was assessed, as well as aspects of the therapeutic alliance (or the degree to which the patient and provider work together toward mutual treatment goals). Findings indicated that telehealth CBT-I is not inferior to the standard of care; face-to-face CBT-I.[28] Initial improvements and 3-month post-treatment outcomes on measures of insomnia severity did not differ between treatment groups. As important, treatment credibility ratings and measures of the therapeutic alliance did not differ between conditions. These findings suggest that in addition to being effective, telehealth CBT-I is a valid and acceptable treatment strategy for insomnia treatment seekers.[28,29]

The dramatic circumstances of the coronavirus disease 2019 (COVID-19) pandemic abruptly disrupted the conventional, in-person model of delivery for most health care services, CBT-I included. With social restrictions and stay-at-home or quarantine orders in place, health care organizations and practices were challenged to pivot to alternative strategies for provision of services. Sleep complaints escalated significantly.[30] High treatment efficacy and acceptability coupled with the inadequate availability of providers spurred an increase in the need for and delivery of telehealth CBT-I. The remainder of this chapter focuses on the delivery of telehealth CBT-I.

Advantages and Challenges of Telehealth CBT-I

Telehealth services in general are well received by both patients and providers.[31] With this, however, there is recognition that the modality of telehealth carries with it both advantages and disadvantages, some of which are specific to telehealth CBT-I and others that are more broadly applicable. These are delineated in Tables 15.1 and 15.2.

Telehealth Visit–Related Responsibilities

The mechanics of the provision of telehealth services are different from those of face-to-face visits, and as such, they deserve attention here. The provider's responsibilities can broadly be categorized

TABLE 15.1 ■ **Advantages of Telehealth CBT-I**

- Allows patients to access expert treatment or insomnia in the comfort of their home environment in a way that can be just as secure and private as face-to-face treatment
- Allows patients to attend treatment sessions without incurring travel time; this results in less time away from work or school, less childcare, and fewer costs to patients
- Reduces driving-related risks for patients with excessive daytime sleepiness
- Reduces issues related to mobility and/or age and may make visit attendance safer and less fatiguing
- Eliminates potential stigma of sitting in the waiting room of a treatment center
- Eliminates issues associated with forgotten sleep diaries and allows providers to more easily access these data
- Allows providers to potentially see the patient's sleeping environment and other relevant aspects of the home environment, which helps personalize recommendations and may help build rapport
- Encourages good listening practices and "turn taking" in conversations because parties cannot speak over one another
- Increases geographic reach of providers of CBT-I, which has been a limiting factor of treatment provision[32]
- Increases the potential number of patients who can receive group treatment by a trained provider via telehealth[29]
- Reduces transportation-related or weather-related issues resulting in fewer late arrivals, no-shows, and cancellations and therefore increases productivity[29]
- Reduces the need for valuable and expensive clinic space and some aspects of overhead for the provider and facility

TABLE 15.2 ■ **Challenges of Telehealth CBT-I**

- May result in a sense of "intrusion" into a patient's home
- May be difficult for patients to find a fully private space
- May result in sessions during which patients are distracted (e.g., conducting a visit while at their workplace, while driving, or while managing home-related or childcare-related tasks)
- May result in reduced satisfaction for patients who prefer face-to-face treatment
- May reduce service provision to populations with more limited access to Wi-Fi and/or necessary devices
- May be more challenging for older adults or cognitively impaired patients to utilize the necessary technology
- May result in lower patient satisfaction or lower productivity if there are connectivity or technical issues during the visit
- May result in potential reimbursement and licensing concerns

as technical considerations, privacy and security concerns, legal and regulatory concerns, licensure and malpractice issues, establishment of emergency protocols, and visit integrity. These responsibilities must be addressed throughout the course of contact with the patient from pre-visit activities through the termination of treatment. Strategies to address many of these responsibilities follow. It is also critical to recognize that the specifics of these responsibilities will be dependent on the practitioner's state of licensure and will also likely vary over time.[33] Providers must familiarize themselves with local regulations. Section II of this text, "Implementation of Telemedicine," provides a comprehensive review of these concerns.

Recommended provider pre-visit activities are as follows[34]:

- Ensure that all electronic devices and programs are approved by the provider's institution for privacy and security.
- Ensure appropriate, non-distracting surroundings and privacy. Minimize clutter and noise in your environment, and ensure that your background appears professional.
- Pre-load any materials needed for the visit in readily available windows, such as sleep diary, sleep education handouts, and polysomnography (PSG) results to review, etc.

- Minimize or close any open windows with sensitive information or information not needed for the appointment.
- Position the camera of your device so you are facing forward while speaking to the patient and are centered on the screen, ensuring good eye contact. Ensure adequate lighting so you are not in a shadow.

Recommended provider start-of-visit activities are as follows[35]:
- Determine the identity and location of the patient (e.g., whether the patient is in a state where the provider is licensed).
- Introduce yourself to the patient, state the purpose of the appointment, and share your relevant credentials.[5]
- Ensure that the patient has privacy and is not distracted (e.g., cooking, driving, answering emails, or working). Consider offering to reschedule if the patient cannot discontinue other activities.
- Create a plan for what to do if either party is disconnected during the visit (e.g., the provider will phone the patient at the preferred contact number, or the patient will attempt to log back onto the visit).

Recommended provider close-of-visit responsibilities are as follows:
- Provide the patient with a phone number or with instructions for how to access the electronic medical record (EMR) portal message center so the patient can contact the office for questions, concerns, or any follow-up needs.
- Share relevant forms, releases of information, handouts, and any patient instructions as appropriate, either via EMR portal message center or secure email.
- Explain how to upload sleep diaries, continuous positive airway pressure (CPAP) data downloads, and wearable sleep data device information via the EMR portal message center or secure email prior to the next visit.
- Close completely out of the session on your device.

Telehealth CBT-I Treatment Specifics

Telemedicine services should be as identical as possible to a live office visit including a thorough assessment, diagnosis, treatment planning, session content, and provision of handouts or other materials.[15]

With this in mind, the tasks of the first visit include building rapport, developing a therapeutic alliance, and setting expectations for therapy. Building rapport is paramount for CBT-I because providers will often need to ask patients to engage in behaviors that may be counterintuitive, novel, or difficult.

This aspect of treatment must be intentional when CBT-I is conducted remotely, and two simple tools may prove helpful: allowing patients to speak about their sleep problems for a short period without interruption at the beginning of the visit and then following up with a question about challenges patients face as a result of these issues.[36,37] Langewitz et al. found that 2 minutes of uninterrupted listening was sufficient for nearly 80% of patients, even those with complex histories, and Ofri noted that questioning patients about the hardest challenges they face due to their presenting problem elicited crucial information efficiently.[36,37]

The provider will also want to set expectations during the first visit by reviewing the typical duration and frequency of CBT-I, the typical content of each visit, the importance of a thorough assessment before treatment is undertaken, and the role of homework in both providing a baseline and tracking sleep data to be able to demonstrate improvement. Visit length is typically 30 to 60 minutes. Assessment and first treatment visits tend to require more time than subsequent visits.

The provider will also need to discuss the need for privacy during telehealth visits and the importance of limiting distractions. Finally, the first visit should provide specific directions for patients, enabling them to use the EMR portal to upload diaries, receive handouts and instructions, and communicate questions or concerns.

ASSESSMENT

Successful CBT-I begins with a thorough assessment of the patient's perception of sleep itself and an assessment of the physical, psychological, behavioral, and environmental factors that influence sleep. Some of this can be accomplished with questionnaires that are made available to the patient prior to the first visit. Commonly used standardized questionnaires include the Pittsburgh Sleep Quality Index, Insomnia Severity Index, Dysfunctional Beliefs and Attitudes about Sleep the Scale, and the Epworth Sleepiness Scale.[38-41] Some EMR systems allow these to be administered to the patient well before the first visit or just before the telemedicine visit begins. The ISI is widely used clinically and in research.

Insomnia Severity Index

Subject ID: _____   Date: _____

For each question below, please circle the number corresponding most accurately to your sleep patterns in the LAST MONTH.

For the first three questions, please rate the SEVERITY of your sleep difficulties.

1. Difficulty falling asleep:

None	Mild	Moderate	Severe	Very Severe
0	1	2	3	4

2. Difficulty staying asleep:

None	Mild	Moderate	Severe	Very Severe
0	1	2	3	4

3. Problem waking up too early in the morning:

None	Mild	Moderate	Severe	Very Severe
0	1	2	3	4

4. How SATISFIED/dissatisfied are you with your current sleep pattern?

Very Satisfied	Satisfied	Neutral	Dissatisfied	Very Dissatisfied
0	1	2	3	4

5. To what extent do you consider your sleep problem to INTERFERE with your daily functioning (e.g., daytime fatigue, ability to function at work/daily chores, concentration, memory, mood).

Not at all interfering	A Little interfering	Somewhat interfering	Much interfering	Very much interfering
0	1	2	3	4

6. How NOTICEABLE to others do you think your sleeping problem is in terms of impairing the quality of your life?

Not at all noticeable	A little noticeable	Somewhat noticeable	Much noticeable	Very much noticeable
0	1	2	3	4

7. How WORRIED/distressed are you about your current sleep problem?

Not at all	A little	Somewhat	Much	Very much
0	1	2	3	4

ISI: © Morin, C.M. (1993 and 1996) ISI-Clinian version: © Morin, C.M. (1993, 1996, 2000, 2006)

There are seven items in the ISI, with each rated on a scale from 0 to 4. The total score is the sum of each individual item and can range from 0 to 28 (28 indicating the most severe insomnia).

Interpretation: Scores between 0 and 7 are considered normal; between 8 and 14 indicate mild to moderate insomnia; between 15 and 21 indicate moderate insomnia; and between 22 and 28 indicate severe insomnia. Scores above 15 suggest that the patient should have evaluation and treatment.

In addition, questionnaires that gather the following information are helpful: onset of sleep difficulties or precipitating events, a full sleep history including any prior sleep study findings, a psychiatric history, a medical history, and a review of current medications including any current and past prescription sleep medications and over-the-counter sleep aids. A mental status examination is conducted at the first visit.

An insomnia intake questionnaire can also be completed prior to the assessment appointment or at the time of assessment. This questionnaire can include items covering weekday and weekend bedtime range, sleep onset latency range, number of night wakings and typical length of each, typical activities during night awakenings, and the usual rise time range. Daytime behaviors that influence sleep such as use of stimulants or napping are noted. The patient's chronotype is also assessed. In addition, if a patient wears a sleep or activity tracker, this information can be collected at this time.

Daily habits are assessed and recorded, specifically, the use of caffeine, nicotine, alcohol, marijuana, or other substances or supplements; exercise habits and usual mealtimes; and whether or not the patient engages in night eating.

Once this basic data has been obtained, the provider can conduct additional assessment with the patient as part of the first visit. The patient's concerns and goals with regard to sleep are elicited. The bedtime routine is documented, noting any rigid bedtime rituals, and the bedroom environment is reviewed in detail with particular attention to temperature, light, noise, and adequacy of the bed and bedding. If the behavior of other family members affects sleep, this is noted as well (e.g., the patient may have young children, a partner with a very different sleep schedule or one whose sleep may be disruptive to the patient, or a household member who requires care at night). Pets and their habits are also reviewed in terms of how these may negatively affect the patient's sleep.

Collateral information from relevant other parties such as partners, parents, or relatives is also very useful. A visual assessment of the sleep environment, if the patient is agreeable, can also provide valuable information. The provider concludes the session by reviewing the baseline sleep diary or sleep tracker procedure (Box 15.1).

Wearable devices are better at detecting sleep than detecting wake, and therefore are less accurate on nights with poor or disrupted sleep, when a patient is lying in bed trying to sleep but still awake.[42] On these nights, a patient's data may indicate that the patient's total sleep time is greater than it actually was. This is because these devices often use an accelerometer to detect movement and a sensor to detect heart rate; lying very still in bed can mimic sleep. Conversely, wearable devices can be misleading in the opposite fashion, leading a patient to believe that sleep was disrupted when, in fact, it was relatively well preserved. Patients have been observed to become invested in the output from their wearables, even when the data contradict their own experiences.[43]

On the positive side, these devices can make collecting sleep diary data easier and more automatic than filling out sleep logs by hand. In addition, they can also be helpful during treatment by tracking some simple sleep metrics (e.g., the range of bedtimes and rise times over a given week or the typical time at night that there is a long nocturnal episode of wakefulness). These devices can be useful for encouraging patients to reduce time in bed (TIB) or helping them be more accountable in terms of whether they are adhering consistently to the bedtimes and rise times agreed upon as part of CBT-I.

BOX 15.1 ■ Sleep Trackers

The use of wearable activity and sleep trackers, or "wearables," is becoming more prevalent. The current models, however, are not entirely accurate in terms of staging sleep (light, deep, and REM) and tend to overestimate sleep and underestimate awakening after sleep onset. However, some of these devices perform as well or better than actigraphy on sleep/wake performance measures.[42]

On the negative side, some patients have a tendency to overanalyze their sleep quality due to these devices. They may find the sleep staging data, for example, to be discouraging if their device shows very little deep sleep, or they may try to achieve high "sleep scores" night after night. It is important to teach patients how to benefit from the data these devices provide without becoming overly influenced by this information. It is also critical to teach them to rely more on the proven techniques of CBT-I (such as maintaining a consistent sleep schedule and keeping their bed associated with sleep only) than on the data and sleep scores these devices provide.

PSG is rarely used in the initial assessment of insomnia; PSG utility is greatest when an underlying sleep disorder is expected or if the patient does not respond to CBT-I.

Concomitant with CBT-I, some patients may need treatment for other disorders including substance use disorders, eating disorders, post-traumatic stress disorder (PTSD), or anxiety and mood disorders including bipolar disorder, as these may interfere with treatment adherence or ability to benefit from therapy.[44] In addition, sometimes CBT-I is deferred until after positive airway pressure (PAP) therapy is initiated if the patient has sleep apnea because PAP therapy often improves sleep maintenance insomnia and reduces early morning awakening.

It should also be noted that CBT-I is not appropriate for all populations, and its implementation may require additional considerations. For example, patients who do not have the cognitive capacity to follow treatment recommendations independently may not benefit from CBT-I. Also, patients with seizure disorders, severe anxiety, and bipolar disorder may require extra consideration and collaboration with the medical team.[44]

TREATMENT COMPONENTS

In the first treatment session, sleep diary data and/or wearable data are reviewed to establish and confirm the patient's baseline sleep parameters. Two weeks of baseline data are typically preferred to allow for the natural variability in nightly sleep.[44] Treatment begins with the two principle components of behavioral sleep treatment, stimulus control and sleep restriction.[45,46] The theory and reasoning behind these treatment strategies are reviewed with the patient.

Stimulus control treatment, first introduced by Bootzin in 1972, rests on operant conditioning principles.[45] Good sleepers, as a result of their history of falling and staying asleep easily, experience the bed and bedroom as a reliable cue for sleep. For poor sleepers, who repeatedly experience lying in bed and not sleeping, the bed and the bedroom become associated with anxiety, agitation, and frustration. The bed and the bedroom become stimuli associated with arousal and wakefulness, which are incompatible with sleep. Stimulus control reassociates the sleep environment with relaxation and sleep.

Patients are given a core set of instructions:
- Use the bed for sleep and sex only.
- Go to bed only when sleepy.
- Get out of bed after a brief period of time when unable to sleep.
- Maintain a consistent rise time.
- Avoid or minimize daytime naps.

Appropriate activities for the time prior to bedtime and while awake during the night are also reviewed.

Sleep restriction therapy, first presented by Spielman and colleagues in 1987, is usually presented at the same time as stimulus control treatment.[46] Sleep restriction aims to enhance sleep drive by creating a condition of intentional sleep deprivation. This is done by limiting TIB in a systematic fashion. Sleep becomes better consolidated, with less time awake during the night.

The first steps in sleep restriction are to determine initial allowable TIB and the window of opportunity for sleep. These are determined based on sleep diary information or wearable data. Total sleep times from the patient's baseline sleep diaries are averaged. This average is used to determine the initial allowable TIB, although patients are not restricted to fewer than 5 or 6 hours in bed regardless of total average time asleep.[47] The target sleep window is largely determined by the patient's habitual or desired rise time. For example, if the patient's rise time is 6:00 AM and the initial recommended total TIB is 6 hours, bedtime is at midnight.

Patients calculate their sleep efficiency (SE) nightly. SE is the ratio of total time asleep divided by total TIB. SE is reviewed on a weekly basis during treatment visits, and TIB is then revised as appropriate.

- If the patient is obtaining an average SE of 85% to 90% in the preceding week, they are allotted 15 to 30 minutes more TIB.
- If SE is 80% to 85% or unchanged in the preceding week, no changes are made.
- If SE is lower than 80%, TIB can be decreased to the average time asleep for the preceding week, not less than 5 to 6 hours, again with the goal of strengthening the homeostatic sleep drive.

Written handouts with guidelines for stimulus control treatment, including suggested appropriate activities for wake time during the night, are provided. Similarly, sleep restriction worksheets are provided to allow patients to calculate their SE. These materials are provided either through secure email or the patient's EMR communication portal.

Sleep compression therapy may be used as an alternative to sleep restriction therapy for patients who may have difficulty with sleep restriction for a variety of reasons (e.g., older patients, patients with daytime fatigue or sleepiness, patients with excessive anxiety about sleep restriction, patients who may react poorly to sudden changes in their sleep schedules); with this technique, TIB is gradually restricted until the TIB closely matches actual total sleep time or when an optimal balance is reached. This sleep compression can be accomplished over several weeks in increments of 20 to 30 minutes per week. In addition, naps are also limited to 30 minutes, completed before 2 PM. Sometimes this more gradual restriction is as successful for patients and also less difficult.[48]

The second treatment session begins with a review of sleep diaries and/or wearable data. TIB is modified as shown earlier based on SE. Adherence concerns are addressed. This session often involves problem-solving issues related to sleep restriction and the window of opportunity for sleep, as well as appropriate bedtime and middle-of-the-night activities related to stimulus control treatment.

Circadian rhythm–related techniques to increase daytime wakefulness and entrain the desired rise time are also outlined. These techniques include obtaining morning sunlight exposure, engaging in light physical activity, seeking social interaction, and having a meal shortly after arising.

Basic sleep hygiene information is presented including the optimal use of caffeine, alcohol, and nicotine. Sleep hygiene also includes recommendations for electronics use to minimize their disruption of sleep, the role of exercise and optimal timing for this, and the importance of choosing appropriate bedtime snacks and avoiding night eating.

Cognitive therapy for dysfunctional beliefs about sleep is initiated. Cognitive restructuring techniques are used.

CBT-I also includes the start of sleep education, which is ongoing throughout treatment. The 3P etiological model of insomnia; sleep-wake regulation including process S and process C; substances that influence sleep including nicotine, caffeine, and recreational drugs; sleep throughout the life cycle; sleep architecture; and the role of exercise are reviewed.

The third treatment session begins with a review of sleep diary and/or wearable data, and adherence challenges are discussed and resolved. Adjustments to TIB are made as appropriate, based on SE. Sleep education includes optimization of the bedtime routine and bedroom environment, such as maintaining a cool, comfortable temperature, establishing a quiet and dark environment, removing clutter, and ensuring that the bed and bedding are adequate and comfortable. Issues relating to family members and the disruptions they may cause to the patient's sleep are addressed directly as these can affect adherence. Relaxation strategies are introduced as needed.

Later CBT-I sessions continue to review and adjust TIB and address adherence as needed. These sessions often include discussions of medication tapering, if desired, after improved sleep skills are acquired.[44,49] Coordination with the prescribing provider is essential.

The final visit for CBT-I addresses relapse prevention. This includes compiling a summary of the techniques and concepts that were helpful for the patient. The provider and the patient also discuss any situations or upcoming events that may temporarily worsen sleep, and plans are made to address these. The patient is reminded that a few nights of poor sleep will not necessarily result in an extended period of insomnia. Relevant research is shared with patients demonstrating that improvements in sleep resulting from CBT-I are likely to be maintained and continue to improve over time.[4] In addition, standardized questionnaires administered at intake can be repeated to demonstrate treatment gains. The patient should also be encouraged to follow up with the provider for additional CBT-I sessions as needed.

Reimbursement and the Practice of Telehealth CBT-I

For telehealth CBT-I to thrive, reimbursement issues must be addressed so insurance service coverage does not become a substantial barrier to patients seeking care.[50] Perrin et al. note that reimbursement issues are far less problematic in the VA health system and have probably resulted in telemedicine's relative success within this system. In addition, a licensed psychologist at a VA medical center can provide services to a veteran in any other state, and this has significantly expanded the ability of veterans to receive the care they need.[50] The acceleration during the pandemic of the provision of CBT-I via telehealth was greatly facilitated by a transition to equivalent reimbursement for this type of service compared with face-to-face services. Federal legislation to make these equivalencies permanent will be critical as will the development and acceptance of interstate practice agreements.[29,50,51]

Conclusion

CBT-I is the practice standard for treating insomnia and can be delivered effectively and efficiently via telehealth. The COVID-19 pandemic has greatly accelerated this high-quality method of delivering CBT-I services. This trend is likely to significantly increase the number and geographic reach of patients who can receive this first-line treatment. A strong therapeutic alliance can be achieved if approached intentionally, even when the treatment visits are conducted remotely. Telehealth CBT-I may offer some advantages not previously available to a provider such as the ability to assess the patient's sleep environment and more easily interact with other people connected to the patient without these parties having to travel to the clinic. Since patients have embraced telehealth services, telehealth CBT-I is likely to continue to expand significantly in the coming years. Evaluation of patient and clinical characteristics to determine who benefits most from telehealth CBT-I are needed to continue to evaluate, refine, and extend our knowledge of best practices.[4,28,51] In addition, outcome studies on patient costs, health-care accessibility, and reimbursement are needed to ensure the viability of telehealth CBT-I moving forward.[51]

References

1. Panel CC. Recommended amount of sleep for a healthy adult: a joint consensus statement of the American Academy of Sleep Medicine and Sleep Research Society. *Sleep*. 2015;38(6):843-844.
2. American Academy of Sleep Medicine. *International Classification of Sleep Disorders: Diagnostic and Coding Manual*. 2005:51-55.
3. American Psychiatric Association. *Diagnostic and Statistical Manual of Mental Disorders: DSM-5*. Washington, DC: American Psychiatric Association; 2013.
4. Edinger JD, Arnedt JT, Bertisch SM, et al. Behavioral and psychological treatments for chronic insomnia disorder in adults: an American Academy of Sleep Medicine systematic review, meta-analysis, and GRADE assessment. *J Clin Sleep Med*. 2021;17(2):263-298.

5. Perlis ML, Jungquist C, Smith MT, Posner D. *Cognitive Behavioral Treatment of Insomnia: A Session-by-Session Guide.* New York, NY: Springer Science & Business Media; 2006.

6. Morin CM, Bootzin RR, Buysse DJ, Edinger JD, Espie CA, Lichstein KL. Psychological and behavioral treatment of insomnia: update of the recent evidence (1998–2004). *Sleep.* 2006;29(11):1398-1414.

7. Trauer JM, Qian MY, Doyle JS, Rajaratnam SM, Cunnington D. Cognitive behavioral therapy for chronic insomnia: a systematic review and meta-analysis. *Ann Intern Med.* 2015;163(3):191-204.

8. Ma Y, Hall DL, Ngo LH, Liu Q, Bain PA, Yeh GY. Efficacy of cognitive behavioral therapy for insomnia in breast cancer: a meta-analysis. *Sleep Med Rev.* 2021;55:101376.

9. Taylor DJ, Pruiksma KE. Cognitive and behavioural therapy for insomnia (CBT-I) in psychiatric populations: a systematic review. *Int Rev Psychiatry.* 2014;26(2):205-213.

10. Qaseem A, Kansagara D, Forciea MA, Cooke M, Denberg TD. Management of chronic insomnia disorder in adults: a clinical practice guideline from the American College of Physicians. *Ann Intern Med.* 2016;165(2):125-133.

11. Riemann D, Baglioni C, Bassetti C, et al. European guideline for the diagnosis and treatment of insomnia. *J Sleep Res.* 2017;26(6):675-700.

12. Schutte-Rodin S, Broch L, Buysse D, Dorsey C, Sateia M. Clinical guideline for the evaluation and management of chronic insomnia in adults. *J Clin Sleep Med.* 2008;4(5):487-504.

13. Morgenthaler T, Kramer M, Alessi C, et al. Practice parameters for the psychological and behavioral treatment of insomnia: an update. An American Academy of Sleep Medicine report. *Sleep.* 2006;29(11):1415-1419.

14. Wilson S, Anderson K, Baldwin D, et al. British Association for Psychopharmacology consensus statement on evidence-based treatment of insomnia, parasomnias and circadian rhythm disorders: an update. *J Psychopharmacol.* 2019;33(8):923-947.

15. Singh J, Badr MS, Diebert W, et al. American Academy of Sleep Medicine (AASM) position paper for the use of telemedicine for the diagnosis and treatment of sleep disorders. *J Clin Sleep Med.* 2015;11(10):1187-1198.

16. Sarmiento KF, Folmer RL, Stepnowsky CJ, et al. National expansion of sleep telemedicine for Veterans: The TeleSleep Program. *J Clin Sleep Med.* 2019;15(9):1355-1364.

17. Ström L, Pettersson R, Andersson G. Internet-based treatment for insomnia: a controlled evaluation. *J Consult Clin Psychol.* 2004;72(1):113-120.

18. Lichstein KL, Scogin F, Thomas SJ, et al. Telehealth cognitive behavior therapy for co-occurring insomnia and depression symptoms in older adults. *J Clin Psychol.* 2013;69(10):1056-1065.

19. van der Zweerde T, Lancee J, Ida Luik A, van Straten A. Internet-delivered cognitive behavioral therapy for insomnia: tailoring cognitive behavioral therapy for insomnia for patients with chronic insomnia. *Sleep Med Clin.* 2020;15(2):117-131.

20. Manber R, Simpson NS, Bootzin RR. A step towards stepped care: Delivery of CBT-I with reduced clinician time. *Sleep Med Rev.* 2015;19:3-5.

21. Espie CA, Emsley R, Kyle SD, et al. Effect of digital cognitive behavioral therapy for insomnia on health, psychological well-being, and sleep-related quality of life: a randomized clinical trial. *JAMA Psychiatry.* 2019;76(1):21-30.

22. Horsch CH, Lancee J, Griffioen-Both F, et al. Mobile phone-delivered cognitive behavioral therapy for insomnia: a randomized waitlist controlled trial. *J Med Internet Res.* 2017;19(4):e70.

23. Zachariae R, Lyby MS, Ritterband LM, O'Toole MS. Efficacy of internet-delivered cognitive-behavioral therapy for insomnia–a systematic review and meta-analysis of randomized controlled trials. *Sleep Med Rev.* 2016;30:1-10.

24. Holmqvist M, Vincent N, Walsh K. Web- vs. telehealth-based delivery of cognitive behavioral therapy for insomnia: a randomized controlled trial. *Sleep Med.* 2014;15(2):187-195.

25. Gehrman P, Shah MT, Miles A, Kuna S, Godleski L. Feasibility of group cognitive-behavioral treatment of insomnia delivered by clinical video telehealth. *Telemed J E Health.* 2016;22(12):1041-1046.

26. Gehrman P, Barilla H, Medvedeva E, et al. Randomized trial of telehealth delivery of cognitive-behavioral treatment for insomnia vs. in-person treatment in veterans with PTSD. *J Affect Disord Rep.* 2020;1:100018.

27. McCarthy MS, Matthews EE, Battaglia C, Meek PM. Feasibility of a telemedicine-delivered cognitive behavioral therapy for insomnia in rural breast cancer survivors. *Oncol Nurs Forum.* 2018;45(5):607-618.

28. Arnedt JT, Conroy DA, Mooney A, et al. Telemedicine versus face-to-face delivery of cognitive behavioral therapy for insomnia: a randomized controlled noninferiority trial. *Sleep.* 2021;44(1):zsaa136.
29. Simpson N, Manber R. Extending the reach of cognitive behavioral therapy for insomnia via telemedicine. *Sleep.* 2021;44(1):zsaa241.
30. Mandelkorn U, Genzer S, Choshen-Hillel S, et al. Escalation of sleep disturbances amid the COVID-19 pandemic: a cross-sectional international study. *J Clin Sleep Med.* 2021;17(1):45-53.
31. Andrews E, Berghofer K, Long J, et al. Satisfaction with the use of telehealth during COVID-19: an integrative review. *Int J Nurs Stud Adv.* 2020;2:100008.
32. Hsieh C, Rezayat T, Zeidler MR. Telemedicine and the management of insomnia. *Sleep Med Clin.* 2020;15(3):383-390.
33. Abrams J, Sossong S, Schwamm LH, et al. Practical issues in delivery of clinician-to-patient telemental health in an academic medical center. *Harv Rev Psychiatry.* 2017;25(3):135-145.
34. Hawaii State Department of Health Genomics Section. Telehealth Best Practices 2020 [updated 3/20/2020]. Available at: https://www.youtube.com/watch?v=zTkTUVCUf9Y. Accessed March 1, 2024.
35. Shore JH, Yellowlees P, Caudill R, et al. Best practices in videoconferencing-based telemental health April 2018. *Telemed J E Health.* 2018;24(11):827-832.
36. Langewitz W, Denz M, Keller A, et al. Spontaneous talking time at start of consultation in outpatient clinic: cohort study. *BMJ.* 2002;325(7366):682-683.
37. Ofri D. *What Patients Say,* What Doctors Hear. Boston: Beacon Press; 2017.
38. Buysse DJ, Reynolds III CF, Monk TH, et al. The Pittsburgh Sleep Quality Index: a new instrument for psychiatric practice and research. *Psychiatry Res.* 1989;28(2):193-213.
39. Bastien CH, Vallières A, Morin CM. Validation of the Insomnia Severity Index as an outcome measure for insomnia research. *Sleep Med.* 2001;2(4):297-307.
40. Johns MW. A new method for measuring daytime sleepiness: the Epworth Sleepiness Scale. *Sleep.* 1991;14(6):540-545.
41. Morin CM. Dysfunctional beliefs and attitudes about sleep: prelim inary scale development and description. The Behavior Therapist. 1994;Summer:163–164. 40.
42. Chinoy ED, Cuellar JA, Huwa KE, et al. Performance of seven consumer sleep-tracking devices compared with polysomnography. *Sleep.* 2021;44(5):zsaa291.
43. Baron KG, Abbott S, Jao N, et al. Orthosomnia: Are some patients taking the quantified self too far? *J Clin Sleep Med.* 2017;13(2):351-354.
44. Manber R, Carney CE. *Treatment Plans and Interventions for Insomnia: A Case Formulation Approach.* New York, NY: Guilford Publications; 2015.
45. Bootzin RR. Stimulus control treatment for insomnia. Proceedings of the 80th Annual meeting of the American Psychological Association. 1972;7:395-396.
46. Spielman AJ, Saskin P, Thorpy MJ. Treatment of chronic insomnia by restriction of time in bed. *Sleep.* 1987;10(1):45-56.
47. Manber R, Friedman L, Siebern AT, et al. *Cognitive Behavioral Therapy for Insomnia in Veterans: Therapist Manual.* Washington, DC: U.S. Department of Veterans Affairs; 2014.
48. Lichstein KL, Riedel BW, Wilson NM, et al. Relaxation and sleep compression for late-life insomnia: a placebo-controlled trial. *J Consult Clin Psychol.* 2001;69(2):227.
49. Hintze JP, Edinger JD. Hypnotic discontinuation in chronic insomnia. *Sleep Med Clin.* 2020;15(2):147-154.
50. Perrin PB, Pierce BS, Elliott TR. COVID-19 and telemedicine: a revolution in healthcare delivery is at hand. *Health Sci Rep.* 2020;3(2):e166.
51. Zia S, Fields BG. Sleep telemedicine: an emerging field's latest frontier. *Chest.* 2016;149(6):1556-1565.

Telemedicine Diagnostics and Management

CHAPTER 16

In-Laboratory Sleep Testing in the Telemedicine Era

Shannon S. Sullivan ■ Therese Santiago

Introduction

In-laboratory sleep testing using telemedicine may seem like a contradiction in terms, but in fact, investigation into "laboratory quality" polysomnography (PSG) in hybrid or out-of-laboratory settings has been ongoing for decades,[1,2] though traditional reimbursement models have not always driven efficient development or scale. Furthermore, real-time monitoring of PSG from a distant site is much less studied than positive airway pressure (PAP) therapy or clinic televisits/teleconsultation. Nonetheless, due to changing considerations and priorities ushered in by the pandemic, the advent of in-laboratory sleep testing using telemedicine is upon the field.

It is important to acknowledge that level I, in-laboratory, technologist-attended monitoring of the patient who is also present in the laboratory is a model that is medically appropriate and necessary in certain circumstances, based on factors such as patient morbidity and disability, presenting symptoms and suspected disorders, medical judgment, and availability of required monitoring tools and data collection systems. However, it is also fair to say that for the workup of some patients and indications for in-laboratory sleep testing, the possibility of development of hybrid-model alternatives to traditional in-laboratory testing may be reasonable.

This chapter will contemplate the essential elements of in-laboratory testing that should be retained in telemedicine-adapted models, evaluate the theoretical requirements needed by telemedicine-supported models for sleep testing, review models relevant to hybrid laboratory-quality data collection, consider how to best identify patients who require in-laboratory testing, and provide evidence for assessing adequacy, outcomes, and scaling for telemedicine-based laboratory-quality sleep testing.

Indications for In-Laboratory Sleep Testing and Requirements for Telemedicine-Enhanced Models

Traditional in-laboratory sleep testing is used to measure physiological functions and changes in sleep-wake [NOT STATE OF SLEEP], and to evaluate for disorders that may be induced by, manifested in, or exhibited by, sleep and/or sleep-wake states. Clinicians may use in-laboratory testing as a tool to evaluate for specific sleep disorders or in some cases, to gauge effectiveness of therapy.[3] The prototypical types of in-laboratory sleep tests performed including overnight PSG, mean sleep latency testing, and maintenance of wakefulness testing, all of which have technical standards and protocols for collection set forth by the American Academy of Sleep Medicine (AASM).[4,5] These tests are used in the diagnostic workup of sleep-related breathing disorders in clinical settings,[6] for example, in patients with significant cardiorespiratory disease, potential respiratory muscle weakness due to a neuromuscular condition, awake hypoventilation or suspicion of sleep-related hypoventilation, chronic opioid medication use, history of stroke or severe insomnia, or in pediatric patients.[7] In-laboratory sleep testing is also used in the evaluation of parasomnias, movement disorders, sleep-related seizures, and hypersomnias such as narcolepsy.

In telemedicine models supporting monitoring and data collection at levels similar to type I testing, the goal is to provide high-quality, real-time monitored, multi-channel data sufficient for diagnostic purposes when the patient, technologist, or both are not in the laboratory together. In contrast with type II testing in which full PSG is performed "at home" without real-time monitoring to assess the quality of data collection and to troubleshoot artifact and lead detachment, type I PSG testing involves attendance by a technologist or other qualified individual[8] in the laboratory with the patient. A recent update to the AASM position statement[9] of the use of telemedicine in the diagnosis and treatment of sleep disorders focuses largely on delivery of clinic visits rather than diagnostic testing per se, but its principles are equally applicable to telemedicine supported models of in-laboratory testing.[10] Table 16.1 outlines selected AASM recommendations for the use of telemedicine in sleep medicine as well as considerations for applications of these principles to sleep testing. Table 16.2 details recent 2021 updates in light of the pandemic experience and highlights the relevance for telemedicine-assisted sleep testing.

As Tables 16.1 and 16.2 indicate, multiple areas of further development are needed to contemplate a scalable telemedicine-assisted or hybrid "sleep laboratory at home" testing experience. Adequate study procedures, including setup and sensor placement; real-time recording and monitoring, including video; adequately addressing and resolving loose leads, artifact, and poor

TABLE 16.1 ■ Select Recommendations for the Use of Telemedicine and Relevance for Sleep Testing

Telemedicine Recommendation	Implications for Telemedicine-Assisted Sleep Testing
Clinical care standards for telemedicine services should mirror those of live visits, including all aspects of diagnosis	• Specific relevant aspects of attended sleep testing should be maintained to support diagnosis (e.g., video, EEG)
Clinical judgment should be exercised when determining the scope and extent of telemedicine applications in diagnosis …of specific patients and sleep disorders.	• Careful consideration of necessary elements of testing based on differential diagnosis, disorders under evaluation, and patient factors
Live interactive telemedicine for sleep disorders, if utilized in a manner consistent with the principles outlined in this document, should be recognized, and reimbursed in a manner competitive or comparable with traditional in-person visits.	• Reimbursement models for remotely set up and monitored testing are largely absent and require development • Investigation into utility is needed
Roles, expectations, and responsibilities of providers involved in the delivery of sleep telemedicine should be defined, including those at originating sites and distant sites.	• For example, in-home setup personnel, remote monitoring technologist, and family members • Protocols for setup and monitoring as well as data integrity, privacy, and security
The practice of telemedicine should aim to promote a care model in which sleep specialists, patients, primary care providers, and other members of the health care team aim to improve the value of health care delivery in a coordinated fashion.	• Understanding patient factors that are best suited to a telemedicine-assisted PSG model • Oversight and responsibility before, during, and after study conduct
Quality assurance processes should be in place for telemedicine care delivery models that aim to capture process measures, patient outcomes, and patient-provider experiences with the model(s) employed.	• Development of quality measures for conduct of telemedicine-assisted models as well as strategies to improve and maintain quality (e.g., diagrams to assist replacement of leads, real-time video help)

EEG, Electroencephalography; *PSG,* polysomnography.
From Singh J, Badr MS, Diebert W, et al. American Academy of Sleep Medicine (AASM) position paper for the use of telemedicine for the diagnosis and treatment of sleep disorders. *J Clin Sleep Med.* 2015;11(10):1187-1198.

TABLE 16.2 ■ 2021 Updated Recommendations for Telemedicine and Relevance for Sleep Testing

Telemedicine Recommendation	Implications for Telemedicine-Assisted Sleep Testing
High-quality, comprehensive sleep care can be provided via telehealth modalities, which are not limited by geographic boundaries.	• Licensing of technologists across geographic boundaries • Differences in scope of practice between states for sleep technologists and respiratory therapists
Synchronous telehealth visits may be performed in lieu of live in-person office visits if they mirror the live visits in quality and process and comply with all licensing, state, federal, and HIPAA regulations for both originating and distant sites, even when both sites are located outside of the traditional office.	• Achieving adequate sensor placement, recording, data quality review, and troubleshooting in real time when the technologist and patient may not be in the same location • Privacy, compliance, and data security requirements
A telemedicine program must maintain a culture of good patient safety encompassing professional accountability, risk assessment, risk management, and infection control, with special consideration for both the physical and psychological safety of the patient at the time of the telemedicine visit.	• Field safety for both the patient and technologist • Adequate infection control practices in the field • Equipment chain of custody
Telehealth may play a vital role in preserving the continuity of sleep health, but advocacy for greater access to telehealth systems to reduce health disparities is needed.	• High-speed, secure Internet access, phone communications • Access to trained technologists with appropriate skill sets
Moving forward, clinical pathways to diagnose and manage sleep disorders are needed to determine the best way to integrate in-person care with telemedicine, including the incorporation of data from sleep-specific and consumer-based technologies.	• Feasibility and usability design and testing • Appropriate patient selection • Establish clinical pathways based on specific disorders, equipment characteristics • Establish reimbursement routes and equity

HIPAA, Health Insurance Portability and Accountability Act.
From Shamim-Uzzaman QA, Bae CJ, Ehsan Z, et al. The use of telemedicine for the diagnosis and treatment of sleep disorders: an American Academy of Sleep Medicine update. J Clin Sleep Med. 2021;17(5):1103-1107.

data quality in real time; and following testing, infection control, and safety protocols, are all necessary components for contemplating telemedicine-assisted sleep testing models. Additionally, anticipating and providing for meeting compliance, privacy, and data security requirements are necessary. Finally, substantial user testing, provision of accessible content (multilingual, appropriate content for visually or hearing-impaired patients), and identifying safe and secure processes for equipment delivery and return are all required.

In-Laboratory Sleep Testing: Lessons Learned From the COVID-19 Pandemic

Over the first 12 months of the coronavirus disease 2019 (COVID-19) pandemic, sleep laboratory operations underwent significant changes. A series of guidelines on the closure and reopening of sleep laboratories were promulgated by various medical societies, recommending the postponement of all non-urgent in-laboratory studies, especially in areas with high COVID-19 transmission.[11-14] These were prompted by efforts to navigate the confusing mix of infection control needs, staff allocation demands, and public health mandates levied during that time. In July 2020, an American Thoracic Society Task Force[11] provided specific guidance for reopening, encompassing conduct of PSGs, with specific consideration of pediatrics, and emphasizing clinical prioritization of patients. It recommended that laboratories start with diagnostic testing at 50% capacity and then open for PAP titrations. It also considered appropriate use of personal protective equipment, nonvented masks and filters, and alternatives such as auto-titrating PAP for sleep-related breathing disorders, even without a diagnostic test, when clinical need demanded it. Even when open, sleep laboratories faced challenges, for example, instituting ventilation updates, instituting additional infection protective measures, and minimizing gathering and crowding. Admission of caregivers during the study was often limited, which made it difficult for those with disabilities or mobility limitations.

Due to such factors, performance of in-laboratory sleep studies ground to a near halt: an estimated 93.6% of sleep centers stopped at least one type of sleep study, and 90.4% stopped or reduced in-laboratory studies by at least 90%.[15] Other reports corroborate the widespread impact of the pandemic on sleep laboratory operations and throughput.[16] At the same time, flexibilities available during the public health emergency allowed provision of care in the absence of PSG, which alleviated the requirement of this documentation to justify therapy.[17] In all, these factors gave rise to a fresh look at the role of in-laboratory sleep testing in diagnosing and treating sleep disorders.[18] Among the concerns raised was that associated clinical features requiring in-laboratory sleep testing, such as heart failure, might also render increased risk for poor outcomes related to COVID-19. With this backdrop, increased use of out-of-center, real-time monitored PSG through telematic data transmission has been predicted.[19]

With respect to breathing disorders, the use of telemedicine for the health consultation and diagnosis of obstructive sleep apnea (OSA) has increased exponentially since the pandemic, as has the desire to develop more convenient, scalable tools for assessment, diagnosis, and treatment follow-up. The availability of pre-existing home sleep apnea test (HSAT) approaches[20] to diagnose OSA alleviated some demand, in particular with the use of disposable HSAT testing devices that take advantage of cloud-based data aggregation and automated scoring. This approach was limited to testing for obstructive sleep-disordered breathing and, while important, did not address more complex breathing disorders, replace in-laboratory testing for therapy requirements, or approach the wide spectrum of other disorders requiring in-laboratory testing. Additionally, although type III HSAT has been well established in the field for a less complicated diagnostic pathway for OSA[6] and was increasingly relied upon in the pandemic,[21] the accuracy and effectiveness of HSAT in diagnosing OSA depends on the brand and the number and type of sensors that are used.[22] Most available HSAT devices do not have sensors that fundamentally measure or reliably and accurately determine sleep-wake state and all sleep stages, such as electroencephalography (EEG), electrooculography (EOG), and electromyography (EMG). Further, the absence of EEG electrodes during home sleep tests can underestimate breathing disorders due to the inability to detect EEG arousals. As such, HSAT has reported a sensitivity of 64% to 100% and a specificity of 41% to 100%.[22] Typically, such devices do not include any measure of carbon dioxide gas exchange, let alone EMG, EEG, video, and other signals required for diagnosis of non-respiratory sleep disorders.

Conducting Laboratory-Quality Testing Remotely: "Tele-Diagnostics"

Among the evolving terminology invoked to convert concepts of telemedicine, two terms are especially relevant. First, *tele-diagnostics* refers to medical diagnosis made by the means of telemedicine, and second, *tele-monitoring* refers to the use of wireless transmission of physiologic or non-invasive data.[23] The telemedicine-augmented equivalent of in-laboratory sleep testing is real-time, at-home monitoring sleep testing; typically envisioned is remotely attended PSG, but the same concepts may be extended to Multiple Sleep Latency Test (MSLT) and Maintenance of

Wakefulness Test (MWT) with additional consideration. Additional terminology has been used to describe such scenarios regarding telemonitored PSG (TM-PSG): *tele-supervision* by a trained sleep technologist and real-time *tele-transmission* of PSG signal and possibly video data from the testing location to the supervising technologist.[24]

Since the pandemic, a renewed interest in updated, telemedicine-assisted level II testing has arisen. Although not physically attended in real time by a technologist, and most likely without video monitoring, it nonetheless provides for the possibility of robust data collection. A decision model in patients with suspected OSA that includes economic analysis has shown that level II testing can be cost-effective and useful to provide the more extensive data provided by PSG, while bypassing the in-laboratory component of the stay.[25] This technology may have a role in evaluation of special populations, for example, people with Down syndrome.[26]

A variant of type II unattended testing with "telemedicine assistance" has also recently been reported among pediatric patients, in which a nurse performed the sensor setup either at the clinic or in the home via a mobile unit, and the child slept at home. Telehealth consultation with a sleep nurse was scheduled just prior to the usual bedtime in the patient's home. The parent was guided through a checklist of all technical aspects of the portable PSG equipment. In the report of 7 years' experience among 233 children (5 to 18 years of age, mean age 10.8 +/− 3.6 years; 28.8% with comorbidities, though neuromuscular disease was excluded), technically successful studies were obtained in 90% (209/233), and 6 hours or more of sleep were obtained in 89.5% of studies.[27] Of note, there were no statistical differences between the quality of studies set up by the mobile sleep team versus the hospital-in-the-home team. Authors concluded that an accurate diagnosis was made in 80% (167/209) of patients, with potential for underestimation in 20% (42/209). Assessment of parental report revealed that 89.3% reported a high-level care, 91% reported increased convenience, and 76% perceived good/excellent telehealth support.

A perhaps closer variant of telemedicine-supported PSG to the traditional type I in-laboratory study is one in which there is real-time monitoring throughout the sleep testing period, either continuously or intermittently, with intervention to fix data collection issues as needed. In such a scenario, the patient may be set up in the clinic or at home, but the sleep testing is conducted at home or any area outside of the sleep laboratory (such as a different monitored environment), while being monitored continuously or at intervals by a trained sleep technologist who is in a different location. An early study on TM-PSG was reported by Gagnadoux et al. in a prospective randomized crossover trial.[28] TM-PSG was conducted in a sleep laboratory and compared with home-based PSG. The TM-PSG was performed in the medical wards of two peripheral hospitals in France, with intermittent, real-time, remote control from the sleep technicians of the central sleep laboratory (every 30 minutes). In case of loss of signal, the technicians instructed the nursing staff at the two hospitals on how to replace the electrodes. The study compared the recordings in terms of interpretable signals from at least one EEG, EOG, EMG, respiratory signals, and arterial oxygen saturation. Among the 99 participants, technical intervention was required for 13 TM-PSG, but nurses could only solve 9 problems. The TM-PSG appeared to have technical advantage with 11% failure rate versus 23% for home PSG, though there was no difference in the PSG index between the home PSG versus the TM-PSG. However, authors concluded that for the context of OSA workup in France, home-based, level II PSG had cost savings.[29]

An additional early investigation into the feasibility of real-time monitoring of at-home PSG reported on 10 fibromyalgia patients who were tested utilizing a 14-channel wearable wireless monitor and a cell-phone–based Gateway system to collect and transfer data.[30] Patients were set up at the physician's office similar to that used in standard in-laboratory testing and then returned home. They were instructed to place the Gateway on a nightstand facing the bed, call the sleep technologist, and have the technologist run a remote desktop program that allowed them to make needed adjustments in real time. Additionally, the technology used in this study did allow for video recordings, which were sent to a remote laboratory and offered real-time functionality to address sensor detachment and make corrective adjustments throughout the night. Authors reported that 1 of the 10 recordings could not be monitored in real time due to lack of cell phone coverage, though data were collected for later review. Furthermore, all 10 subjects had scorable data collected, and the authors note that problem solving such as altering camera position was easily achieved. This study uniquely used video monitoring for setup purposes but did not investigate the possibility of all-night recordings.

In a study of real-time monitored home-based PSG with "telematic data transmission" for the diagnosis of OSA, a 21-subject study in Belgium evaluated results of periodic technician-monitoring of PSG. An additional tool called Sleepbox tool (Sleepbox, Medatec, Belgium) was added to the PSG equipment to transmit recordings to the technicians located at the sleep laboratory in real time (Figure 16.1).[31] They performed remote monitoring of the home PSG every hour. In case of sensor loss, the technician was able to call the patient through Skype or through the microphone of the Sleepbox to ask the patient to replace the sensors. This resulted in 90% of the recordings being evaluated as "good-quality." The two failed recordings consisted of one study with battery failure and one with a poor-quality recording.

Similar to the report by Gagnadoux et al., a prospective observational study on 27 patients admitted to the coronary care unit for acute coronary syndrome was assessed for OSA.[32] One-night PSG was performed within 72 hours of admission while the patients were in the coronary care unit. The study was continuously supervised remotely in real time by sleep technologists from the sleep laboratory, which was in another building of the same hospital, and the sensors were placed by sleep-trained physicians. The Sleepbox was used for transmission, and nurses were trained on how to replace sensors and electrodes when faulty signals were detected. The study showed 100% interpretable sleep recordings. In terms of quality of the recordings for

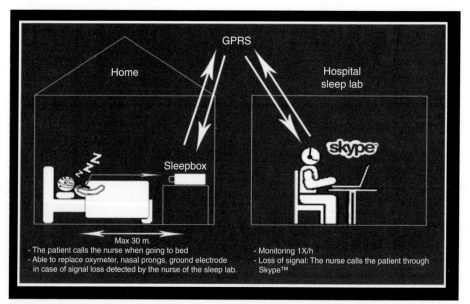

Figure 16.1   Example of Real-Time Monitoring During Polysomnography. A working telemonitoring protocol for out-of-center, monitored polysomnographic recording. *(From Bruyneel M, Van den Broecke S, Libert W, et al. Real-time attended home-polysomnography with telematic data transmission. Int J Med Inform. 2013;82[8]:696-701.)*

PSG, 89% (24/27) of recordings were graded as excellent, and the other 3 were very good or fair. Overall, a total of 10 interventions across the study group were needed by a sleep technologist. In eight cases, this was for the purpose of replacement of the nasal cannula: one for the pulse oximeter and one for electrode repositioning. The median interval between remote detection and the corresponding intervention was 11 minutes. Importantly, the authors noted that six patients were not monitored due to 3G network connection problems, decreasing the efficiency of the Sleepbox to 78%. Nonetheless, the study demonstrates that remote-attended PSG may be feasible in settings among patients with acute medical conditions, especially after connectivity issues are addressed.

Finally, a Spanish study evaluating virtual sleep recording created a "Virtual Sleep Unit" located 80 km from the central sleep laboratory.[33] This study evaluated the performance of real-time monitoring of home-based PSG among patients suspected of having OSA. Placement of leads was performed by the local nursing staff under remote supervision from the central sleep laboratory. During PSG, patients were continuously supervised through tele-monitoring in real time by video using a webcam. There were no polygraph failures observed. There was, however, a 2.5% failure in the data transmission of the recordings.

Although these studies demonstrate feasibility and suggest the potential for scalability,[34] they are limited investigations that cannot fully address the place of TM-PSG in practice. Among the limitations of available evidence, there is an almost complete focus on assessment of such modalities for diagnostic evaluation of sleep-disordered breathing. That said, few of these reports include data on sensors to estimate arterial carbon dioxide tension, which can be an important indicator of alveolar hypoventilation. Such sensors have been successfully used in home-based sleep-related monitoring for over a decade.[15,17] Additionally, use of telemedicine-monitored PSG for diagnostic workup of other key sleep disorders (rapid eye movement [REM] sleep behavior disorder, periodic limb movement disorder, and sleep-related seizures are just a few non-respiratory sleep disorders for which PSG is useful) does not have an evidence base as of yet. Moreover, while real time monitoring of signals collected in real time is feasible, these studies do not report extensively on video monitoring in the home, which is an important aspect of understanding the presentation and manifestation of certain sleep disorders. Video monitoring and recording may become more commonly used as Internet networks are bolstered and data transmission is reliable and robust enough to support such recording. Nonetheless, as of this writing, telemonitored full PSG and its requirements, limitations, and applications are not fully studied and not regularly applied in routine clinical practice.

Advantages, Disadvantages, and Unknowns for Tele-monitoring-Enhanced Sleep Studies

TM-PSG holds promise to address the disadvantages of type III home recordings, while providing potentially scalable alternatives to long wait times and limited availability of and geographic distance to limited sleep center beds[24]; it may also be a scalable future solution when sleep center services are disrupted, for example, for infection control or staffing issues, if robust contactless and remote setup options are developed. This approach may also be more amenable to those who have difficulty traveling, leaving their homes, missing work, or paying for transportation. Because of the wide use of telehealth services during the pandemic, more individuals may be familiar with the use of telehealth services, and more interest in innovation in this space has developed, which may serve to improve the quality of remotely monitored sleep testing. Given the estimated worldwide prevalence of sleep-disordered breathing[35] alone, scalable additional pathways that can take advantage of improvements in technology and the "Internet grid" to meet the variety of clinical needs of patients require development. In terms of cost, studies evaluating potential costs and savings are needed, especially considering recouped workdays; childcare or elder care costs avoided; roundtrip travel costs saved by remote, TM-PSG; and traditional staffing and equipment costs.

There are disadvantages to consider. The shortage of sleep-trained technologists available to set up and conduct real-time attended monitoring remains an issue, as does the availability of means to immediately address technical failures such as poor signals and dislodged sensors or cannulas. Additionally, reliance on potentially weak or unsecure local Internet networks is a substantial potential vulnerability. Like any clinical recording performed remotely and requiring transmission of data, there is the potential for data loss; estimates may approach 4.7% to 20% in some cases.[24] The limitations of geographic location, staffing shortages, and infection control considerations are not necessarily mitigated by telemedicine-assisted sleep studies. The use of telemedicine-monitored PSG for the diagnostic workup of many other key sleep disorders requiring real-time video monitoring and high-quality EMG, EOG, EEG, and other signals does not yet have an evidence base or techniques devoted to development of such expansion. As mentioned earlier, there is little evidence regarding how to adequately conduct telemedicine-supported MSLT or MWT, which have precise protocols, in settings that are fully monitored but remote from the laboratory. Finally, such approaches do not consider what has been termed the *digital divide*,[36] and there is a real risk for increasing health inequalities if access to a facility with secure, high-speed technology excludes those individuals at greatest risk. Finally, models to pay for such services are uncertain and undeveloped, and cost sustainability is fully untested.

Conclusions

Continued advances in technology, including sensor technologies, video and recording possibilities, and high-speed data access, may converge to bring real-time remotely monitored sleep testing into practice. During the pandemic, there has been a greater push in the field to be able to be nimbler in supporting patients with all sleep disorders, not just OSA. These developments allow for further consideration of leveraging availability and advances in technology to accomplish real-time assistance and monitoring of diagnostic testing in sleep. Such telemedicine-assisted models could theoretically expand sleep testing access while achieving reliable results safely. Nonetheless, much more investigation into elements of testing itself, its place in the diagnostic pathways of specific sleep disorders, appropriate patient selection, reimbursement and sustainability models, and clinical protocols to ensure safety, privacy, compliance, and quality remain to be developed.

References

1. Kristo DA, Eliasson AH, Poropatich RK, et al. Telemedicine in the sleep laboratory: feasibility and economic advantages of polysomnograms transferred online. *Telemed J E Health*. 2001;7:219-224.
2. Kayyali HA, Weimer S, Frederick C, et al. Remotely attended home monitoring of sleep disorders. *Telemed J E Health*. 2008;14(4):371-374.
3. Caples SM, Anderson WM, Calero K, et al. Use of polysomnography and home sleep apnea tests for the longitudinal management of obstructive sleep apnea in adults: an American Academy of Sleep Medicine clinical guidance statement. *J Clin Sleep Med*. 2021;17(6):1287-1293.
4. American Academy of Sleep Medicine. *The AASM Manual for the Scoring of Sleep and Associated Events: Rules*, Terminology and Technical Specifications. Version 2.6. Westchester, IL: 2020.
5. Krahn LE, Arand DL, Avidan AY, et al. Recommended protocols for the multiple sleep latency test and the maintenance of wakefulness test in adults: guidance from the American Academy of Sleep Medicine. *J Clin Sleep Med*. 2021;17(12):2489-2498.
6. Kapur VK, Auckley DH, Chowdhuri S, et al. Clinical practice guideline for diagnostic testing for adult obstructive sleep apnea: an American Academy of Sleep Medicine Clinical Practice Guideline. *J Clin Sleep Med*. 2017;13(3):479-504.
7. Kirk V, Baughn J, D'Andrea L, et al. American Academy of Sleep Medicine position paper for the use of a home sleep apnea test for the diagnosis of OSA in children. *J Clin Sleep Med*. 2017;13(10):1199-1203.

8. Polysomnography and sleep testing. CMS.gov Centers for Medicare & Medicaid Services. (n.d.). Available at: https://www.cms.gov/medicare-coverage-database/view/lcd.aspx?lcdId=33405&ver=25, Accessed January 9, 2024.

9. Singh J, Badr MS, Diebert W, et al. American Academy of Sleep Medicine (AASM) position paper for the use of telemedicine for the diagnosis and treatment of sleep disorders. *J Clin Sleep Med.* 2015;11(10):1187-1198.

10. Shamim-Uzzaman QA, Bae CJ, Ehsan Z, et al. The use of telemedicine for the diagnosis and treatment of sleep disorders: an American Academy of Sleep Medicine update. *J Clin Sleep Med.* 2021;17(5):1103-1107.

11. Wilson KC, Kaminsky DA, Michaud G, et al. Restoring pulmonary and sleep services as the COVID-19 pandemic lessens. From an Association of Pulmonary, Critical Care, and Sleep Division Directors and American Thoracic Society-coordinated Task Force. *Ann Am Thorac Soc.* 2020;17(11):1343-1351.

12. Schiza S, Simonds A, Randerath W, et al. Sleep laboratories reopening and COVID-19: a European perspective. *Eur Respir J.* 2021;57:2002722.

13. Ayas NT, Fraser KL, Giannouli E, et al. Helping Canadian health care providers to optimize Sleep Disordered Breathing management for their patients during the COVID-19 pandemic, *Can J Resp Crit Care Sleep Med.* 2020;4(2):81-82, DOI: 10.1080/24745332.2020.1758442

14. Summary of CDC recommendations relevant for sleep practices during Covid-19. American Academy of Sleep Medicine – Association for Sleep Clinicians and Researchers. (Updated January 18, 2021). Available at: https://aasm.org/covid-19-mitigation-strategies-sleep-clinics-labs/. Accessed January 9, 2024.

15. Johnson KG, Sullivan SS, Nti A, et al. The impact of the COVID-19 pandemic on sleep medicine practices. *J Clin Sleep Med.* 2021;17(1):79-87.

16. Kim SW, Kim HH, Kim KY, et al. Impacts of the COVID-19 pandemic on sleep center operations and sleep apnea treatment in Korea: a multicenter survey. *Medicine (Baltimore).* 2021;100(51):e28461.

17. Centers for Medicare and Medicaid Services. *Medicare Telemedicine Health Care Provider Fact Sheet.* Medicare Coverage and Payment of Virtual Services. March 17, 2020. Available at: https://www.cms.gov/newsroom/fact-sheets/medicare-telemedicine-health-care-provider-fact-sheet. Accessed March 1, 2024.

18. Patel SR, Donovan LM. The COVID-19 pandemic presents an opportunity to reassess the value of polysomnography. *Am J Respir Crit Care Med.* 2020;202(3):309-310.

19. Franceschini CM, Smurra MV. Telemedicine in sleep-related breathing disorders and treatment with positive airway pressure devices. Learnings from SARS-CoV-2 pandemic times. *Sleep Sci.* 2022;15(1):118-127.

20. Collop NA, Anderson WM, Boehlecke B, et al. Clinical guidelines for the use of unattended portable monitors in the diagnosis of obstructive sleep apnea in adult patients. Portable Monitoring Task Force of the American Academy of Sleep Medicine. *J Clin Sleep Med.* 2007;3(7):737-747.

21. Gupta M, Ish P, Chakrabarti S, et al. Diagnostic accuracy and feasibility of portable sleep monitoring in patients with obstructive sleep apnea: re-exploring the utility in the current COVID-19 pandemic. *Monaldi Arch Chest Dis.* 2021;92(1):10.4081/monaldi.2021.1818.

22. Qaseem A, Dallas P, Owens DK, et al. Diagnosis of obstructive sleep apnea in adults: a clinical practice guideline from the American College of Physicians. *Ann Intern Med.* 2014;161(3):210-220.

23. Bruyneel M. Telemedicine in the diagnosis and treatment of sleep apnoea. *Eur Respir Rev.* 2019;28(151):180093.

24. Verbraecken J. Telemedicine in sleep-disordered breathing: expanding the horizons. *Sleep Med Clin.* 2021;16(3):417-445.

25. Ayas NT, Jen R, Baumann B. Revisiting level II sleep studies in the era of COVID-19: a theoretical economic decision model in patients with suspected obstructive sleep apnea. *Sleep Sci Pract.* 2021;5(1):11.

26. Cielo CM, Kelly A, Xanthopoulos M, et al. Feasibility and performance of home sleep apnea testing in youth with Down syndrome. *J Clin Sleep Med.* 2023;19(9):1605-1613.

27. Griffiths A, Mukushi A, Adams AM. Telehealth-supported level 2 pediatric home polysomnography. *J Clin Sleep Med.* 2022;18(7):1815-1821.

28. Gagnadoux F, Pelletier-Fleury N, Philippe C, et al. Home unattended versus hospital telemonitored polysomnography in suspected obstructive sleep apnea syndrome: a randomized crossover trial. *Chest.* 2002;121(3):753-758.

29. Pelletier-Fleury N, Gagnadoux F, Philippe C, et al. A cost-minimization study of telemedicine. The case of telemonitored polysomnography to diagnose obstructive sleep apnea syndrome. *Int J Technol Assess Health Care.* 2001;17(4):604-611.

30. Kayyali HA, Weimer S, Frederick C, et al. Remotely attended home monitoring of sleep disorders. *Telemed J E Health*. 2008;14(4):371-374.

31. Bruyneel M, Van den Broecke S, Libert W, et al. Real-time attended home-polysomnography with telematic data transmission. *Int J Med Inform*. 2013;82(8):696-701.

32. Van den Broecke S, Jobard O, Montalescot G, et al. Very early screening for sleep-disordered breathing in acute coronary syndrome in patients without acute heart failure. *Sleep Med*. 2014;15:1539-1546.

33. Coma-Del-Corral MJ, Alonso-Alvarez ML, Allende M, et al. Reliability of telemedicine in the diagnosis and treatment of sleep apnea syndrome. *Telemed J E Health*. 2013;19:7-12.

34. Bruyneel M. Technical developments and clinical use of telemedicine in sleep medicine. *J Clin Med*. 2016;5(12):116.

35. Benjafield AV, Ayas NT, Eastwood PR, et al. Estimation of the global prevalence and burden of obstructive sleep apnoea: a literature-based analysis. *Lancet Respir Med*. 2019;7(8):687-698.

36. Pinnock H, Murphie P, Vogiatzis I, Poberezhets V. Telemedicine and virtual respiratory care in the era of COVID-19. *ERJ Open Res*. 2022;8(3):00111-2022.

37. Bauman KA, Kurili A, Schmidt SL, et al. Home-based overnight transcutaneous capnography/pulse oximetry for diagnosing nocturnal hypoventilation associated with neuromuscular disorders. *Arch Phys Med Rehabil*. 2013;94(1):46-52.

38. Nardi J, Prigent H, Adala A, et al. Nocturnal oximetry and transcutaneous carbon dioxide in home-ventilated neuromuscular patients. *Respir Care*. 2012;57(9):1425-1430.

39. Voulgaris A, Antoniadou M, Agrafiotis M, Steiropoulos P. Respiratory involvement in patients with neuromuscular diseases: a narrative review. *Pulm Med*. 2019;2019:2734054.

CHAPTER 17

Home Sleep Testing

Thomas Penzel

Home Sleep Testing in Sleep Telemedicine

Monitoring of physiological sleep variables in the home setting was done well before the major uptake of telemedicine during the coronavirus disease 2019 (COVID-19) pandemic (see Chapter 2). Thus most clinics did not have any difficulty transitioning into telemedicine because most were already performing the most widely used diagnostic test in the field. Now that the pandemic emergency is over, clinics must ensure that they abide by local regulations as well as ethical standards (see Chapter 3) including informed consent (see Chapter 8), and they must be able to communicate effectively (see Chapters 9 and 10). Reimbursement for sleep telemedicine services has changed and will change in the future (see Chapter 4). Before a home sleep test is considered, an evaluation is required (see Chapter 11).

Overview and Background

Home sleep testing refers to portable monitoring for diagnosing sleep-disordered breathing. The term was introduced in the past decade. In 2014, a National Library of Medicine (NLM) PubMed database search for "home sleep testing" in all fields found 19 publications, and the same search in 2020 returned 83 publications. In mid-2023, the same search resulted in 125 publications. The most recent publications show increased use of home sleep testing instead of in-laboratory testing because the former reduces direct contact between patients and medical staff—an outcome of the impact of the COVID-19 pandemic on medical practice.[1]

The reference method for diagnosing sleep-disordered breathing remains to be cardiorespiratory polysomnography. The recording technology and the scoring criteria used in home sleep testing are derived from this modality. In July 2015, the American Academy of Sleep Medicine (AASM) manual for recording and scoring sleep and associated events added a chapter concerning home sleep apnea testing (version 2.2). Considerable evidence indicates that home sleep testing for sleep-disordered breathing can be as specific and as reliable as sleep laboratory-based polysomnography recordings[2-4] in properly referred patients. Adequate data are available to clinically validate the use of home sleep testing, although it has certain limitations.[5] A workshop consensus report presented the view of the participating medical societies (American Thoracic Society, AASM, American College of Chest Physicians, European Respiratory Society) on using this diagnostic procedure and provided directions for further research.[6] A clinical practice guideline from the American College of Physicians recommends portable sleep monitors for diagnostic testing in patients suspected of having obstructive sleep apnea without severe comorbidity and as an alternative to an in-laboratory sleep study when polysomnography is unavailable.[7] In Europe, home sleep testing has been widely used to diagnose sleep-disordered breathing for several decades.[8]

Guidelines and recommendations for home sleep testing are partially evidence-based. It is essential, however, to critically examine the underlying samples used for evidence evaluation. The clinical validation studies were performed at sleep centers on their patients; consequently, the sample consists of the clinical populations available in sleep centers.[9,10] Clinical populations differ from the general population in that the patients have been referred for evaluation for suspected sleep disorders. This selection leads to a high pretest probability for sleep disorders, and for sleep apnea in particular.[2,11] Factors associated with this increased pretest probability include various physical examination measures and complaints reported by the patient or the bed partner, as follows:

- Loud and irregular snoring
- Observed or reported nocturnal cessation of breathing
- Excessive daytime sleepiness
- Non-specific mental problems such as fatigue, low performance, or cognitive impairment
- Movements during sleep
- Morning dizziness, general headache, dry mouth
- Impaired sexual function
- Obesity
- Arterial hypertension and cardiac arrhythmias

Some of these signs and symptoms are incorporated into sleep apnea screening questionnaires. Clinicians commonly use validated questionnaires in conjunction with home sleep testing to confirm the suspected diagnosis.[12]

As revealed in a literature search, published reports fall into several categories. Some papers describe new devices and compare them with polysomnography. Although reviews of data on existing devices are scarce, they do exist and provide categories for evaluation.[5] These categories are sleep, cardiovascular, oxygen saturation, position, respiratory effort, and flow—the SCOPER acronym. Sensors and systems are evaluated using these categories. Most published studies, however, focus on the role of home sleep testing in sleep apnea diagnosis. Some reports concentrate on the general management of patients with sleep apnea, whereas others focus on home sleep testing. A recent update on the screening for obstructive sleep apnea in adults by the U.S. Preventive Services Task Force considers home sleep testing because of the increasing number of home sleep studies performed.[13] A clear advantage is that recording takes place in the natural home setting, allowing the option to record more than one night and cover the night-to-night variability in sleep-disordered breathing.[14] Presented next is a short technical overview of available systems, followed by a discussion of home sleep testing with respect to requirements and special considerations.

Home Sleep Testing With Four- to Six-Channel Systems for Diagnosing Sleep-Disordered Breathing

Systems for diagnosing sleep-disordered breathing generally fall into one of four classifications defined in an American Sleep Disorders Association (ASDA) standard of practice guideline:[15]

- Level I: attended cardiorespiratory polysomnography with at least seven signals
- Level II: cardiorespiratory polysomnography at home with at least seven signals, unattended
- Level III: unattended portable sleep apnea testing with at least four signals including airflow, respiratory effort, oxygen saturation, electrocardiogram (ECG), or heart rate or pulse rate
- Level IV: unattended one or two signal recordings, such as actigraphy or oximetry

Most diagnostic systems for home sleep testing attain level III device status and record four to six physiological signals but do not record the electroencephalogram (EEG). Evidence-based home sleep testing reviews commissioned by health technology assessment agencies[13,3] revealed limited reliability in the past. More recent studies with recording systems currently in use showed substantial improvement.[10,16] If systems incorporate a thoughtful selection of physiological measures, good signal acquisition, and robust signal-processing techniques, the number of false-positive diagnoses is low.[2] When studies sampling from the general population are compared with studies using clinical populations, the importance of a high pretest probability becomes clear. A high pretest probability reduces the number of false-positive diagnoses. Nonetheless, the overall test specificity is high enough to conclude that home sleep testing for sleep apnea can be recommended under certain conditions[5,7]:

1. Systems should be used only by certified sleep physicians based in certified sleep centers. This recommendation attempts to improve quality control and quality assurance. An interview of the patient and an assessment of complaints should be conducted before performing home sleep testing. This process increases the pretest probability, as explained earlier.
2. Home sleep testing for obstructive sleep apnea is recommended when no other comorbid pulmonary, cardiovascular, mental, neurological, or neuromuscular disorder, heart failure, or other sleep disorder is present. Other sleep disorders to rule out include central sleep apnea, periodic limb movement disorder, insomnia, circadian sleep-wake disorders, and narcolepsy.
3. Some home sleep testing systems can now distinguish between central and obstructive sleep apnea events.
4. Home sleep testing for diagnosing sleep apnea must record oronasal airflow (using a thermistor or nasal pressure sensor); respiratory effort (using inductive plethysmography); oxygen saturation (with a short averaging period over a few [3 to 6] pulses); pulse or heart rate; and body position.
5. Evaluation of the recordings should incorporate visual scoring of respiratory events using the same rules specified for polysomnography.[17,18] (Of course, using the same rules is impossible without the EEG. As a modest proposal to overcome this limitation, Centers for Medicare & Medicaid Services [CMS] rules require a 4% oxyhemoglobin desaturation). Editing of recorded events is necessary to remove artifacts occurring during the recording period. Furthermore, the visual scoring should be performed by trained personnel.
6. The technical specifications and sampling rates for the digital recording should be the same as specified in the evidence-based recommendation for cardiorespiratory polysomnography.[18]

Today, many devices meet level III device criteria. Such home sleep testing devices include pulse oximetry technology to record oxygen saturation and pulse rate. Many systems record oronasal airflow, which reflects intranasal pressure. Few systems still use thermistors for flow recording. Most devices record respiratory effort using either piezo sensors or respiratory inductive plethysmography. Some devices use one belt for rib cage movements, whereas others use two belts (for recording abdominal movements as well). Most systems record body position to identify positional apnea. Few systems record the raw ECG, but many report heart rate derived by other means (e.g., pulse wave). Several systems offer specific options to record signals in sleep apnea patients under therapy. The options are recording continuous positive airway pressure (CPAP) in addition or as an alternative to other airflow signals. The signal will be split into a CPAP reading, corresponding to the set pressure level, and to a respiratory flow reading, which may be observed superposed to the CPAP set. This may vary depending on pressure mode selection (e.g., bilevel or flex modes). This option is essential for using home sleep testing for treatment follow-up studies. Some systems allow an option for recording additional electromyogram (EMG) tibialis activity to detect leg movements; thus far, however, no systematic studies on the utility of this option have been conducted.

Whether home sleep testing can reliably diagnose periodic limb movement disorder remains an open question. Similarly, a few systems can add EEG channels for recording the sleep EEG. Still, no systematic studies have evaluated this option for its potential added diagnostic value for other sleep disorders such as insomnia or hypersomnia. Nonetheless, many systems have been validated for clinical use with their basic signal setup and scoring and analysis software. In general, most systems show good performance, with some minor differences. No overall preference for one or another system emerges from published studies.

Home Sleep Testing With One- to Three-Channel Systems for Diagnosing Sleep-Disordered Breathing

Systematic reviews of home sleep testing for diagnosing sleep-disordered breathing have revealed that systems with one to three channels (pulse oximetry, long-term ECG, actigraphy, and oronasal airflow) are not suitable for routine diagnostic use. Specifically, these devices yield too many false-negative and false-positive results, as reported by Collop and associates[2] and in a more recent systematic review using the new SCOPER criteria.[5] Therefore the application of these devices is not recommended for definitive diagnostic testing for obstructive sleep apnea or to exclude the presence of obstructive sleep apnea.

Some of these devices, however, provide results in patients with severe sleep apnea that suggest sleep-disordered breathing. Therefore high-quality recordings achieved with validated systems of this category can be used to increase the pretest probability before the performance of cardiorespiratory polysomnography or even before four- to six-channel home sleep testing for sleep apnea.

Many technical innovations are currently emerging in this category of devices. A major challenge has been the development of one- to three-channel devices that perform well and can diagnose sleep-disordered breathing. If reliable, such devices could facilitate diagnosis in new patient groups and provide tools for clinicians trained in other specialties with only basic knowledge of sleep medicine. Before initiation of therapy for sleep breathing disorders, however, a physician with a solid background in sleep-disordered breathing who is very familiar with the different treatment options should review the case.[8]

Described next are technologies applicable with both one- to three-channel systems and four- to six-channel diagnostic devices.

New Methods for Home Sleep Testing

Different approaches are being explored for diagnosing sleep-disordered breathing. Some approaches focus on developing new sensors to assess respiration to detect breathing disturbances at night. Other technologies concentrate on evaluating the patient's cardiovascular risk or sleep pathophysiology. In view of the COVID-19 pandemic, some home sleep testing devices were redesigned to be single-use devices, to be applied only once, then transfer the recordings using network infrastructure (telemedicine), while other patient communication is done using video-conferencing.

Assessment of Respiration

Several new sensors use surrogate signals to derive respiratory effort non-invasively. Some of these devices try to derive respiratory measures from direct respiration-related signals. These systems and concepts are discussed next.

A first-line approach entails recording respiratory airflow at the nose and the mouth. Usually, these recordings are accompanied by pulse oximetry to determine oxyhemoglobin saturation. These simple screening devices provide a straightforward analysis for respiratory cessations. They even may distinguish obstructive from central respiratory events by analysis of flow limitation. Problems with obstructed nostrils, partial breathing through the mouth, blocked air tubes, and various artifacts pose logistical challenges to differentiating among the different types of apnea. Nevertheless, good validation studies are available,[20,19] with some limitations.

One approach tries to analyze respiratory sounds from the chest, with the goal of less obtrusive measures for the detection of increased respiratory effort.[21] In other systems, respiratory sounds are recorded at the throat, and signal processing separates cardiac and movement signals first from breathing sounds and snoring. Together with oximetry, such recording quantifies respiratory measures, and snoring is tracked to detect respiratory cessations.[22,23]

Another approach involves recording midsagittal jaw movements based on magnetic distance determination.[24] A magnetic sensor is placed on the chin and another on the forehead to allow continuous determination of relative jaw movements. From this setup, it is possible to derive respiration and snoring. Analysis of this information is then used to detect respiratory events to diagnose sleep apnea.[25] By further analysis, a sleep wakefulness profile may potentially be estimated.[26] Combined with pulse oximetry and perhaps a cardiovascular parameter, this magnetic sensor–jaw movement detection feature is both simple and promising for clinical usefulness.[27]

Pulse Wave Analysis

Many systems try to exploit the pulse wave on the finger or other peripheral sites. Such systems derive parameters from the pulse wave to assess cardiovascular event risk. The pressure wave may be detected with the photoplethysmograph already placed to measure oxygen saturation. In principle, this can be used to detect all forms of respiratory events[28] and cardiovascular event risk as associated with sleep apnea.[29]

Peripheral arterial tonometry (PAT)[30] can be used to assess cardiovascular risk by measuring endothelial function during sleep-disordered breathing episodes. Sympathetic activating events (sometimes referred to as *autonomic arousals*) terminating sleep apnea events are accompanied by attenuated pulse amplitude. This decrease is due to peripheral vasoconstriction caused by sympathetic tone activation. If pulse rate also is analyzed, non-linear biosignal analysis can be used to distinguish between slow wave sleep and rapid eye movement (REM) sleep.[31,32] Several validation studies were published on the use of the Watch-PAT, based on peripheral arterial tonometry, in patients with sleep apnea, with very good results.[19,33] A meta-analysis for this methodology is available and substantiates the diagnostic value of this device, even though it does not incorporate proximal sensors for effort and flow to record respiration, as recommended.[34]

Assessment of Electrocardiographic and Heart Rate Variability Parameters

ECG-derived respiratory parameters are very attractive for simple detection of sleep apnea owing to low costs and wide availability (e.g., Holter ECG software add-on packages, pacemaker ECG analysis add-on packages). To detect sleep apnea from the ECG alone does not require additional electrodes or additional hardware. The respiratory information is derived entirely from analytical software. This kind of analysis also could be performed retrospectively using previously recorded data. Sleep apnea is accompanied by a cyclic variation of heart rate, as already described many years ago.[35] Periodic changes in heart rate are related to the changes in sympathetic tone with apnea events.[36] Modern analysis of heart rate variability can satisfactorily derive cyclic variations of heart rate.[37,38] In addition, the morphology of the ECG wave itself is modulated by respiration. The derived respiratory curve—*ECG-derived respiration*[39]— correlates with respiratory effort and thus can be used to detect sleep-disordered breathing.[28,40] By combining ECG-derived respiration and sleep apnea–related heart rate variability, sleep apnea detection is possible.[37,40,41]

Electrocardiographic and Oximetry Assessments

A number of devices that use the ECG analysis techniques mentioned previously also try to link this approach to previous techniques. Early on, pulse oximetry was applied (with limited success) for portable diagnosis of sleep apnea. Pulse oximetry alone has large diagnostic limitations in patients with arrhythmias or with additional lung diseases such as chronic obstructive pulmonary disease. Combining ECG-based sleep apnea analysis and oximetry is therefore a very promising approach.[42] An early study using pulse rate in addition to oximetry[43] could show that this improves the detection of sleep apnea. One retrospective study showed the advantage over pulse oximetry alone when combined with ECG analysis.[44] In this study, the ECG from a parallel polysomnography recording was evaluated. Based on these results, a combined long-term ECG recording system with oximetry was tested prospectively and provided very convincing results in terms of sleep apnea detection.[42]

Management of Home Sleep Testing in a Sleep Center Setting

Many new studies show high reliability of home sleep testing in detecting sleep apnea.[20] A number of open research questions needing clarification concerning the conditions and restrictions for using home testing are now being addressed in recent studies.[1,2,6] The important parameters are no longer technical limitations, but often study limitations involve selection and/or incorporation bias. The inherent screening process corresponds with the characteristic high pretest probability of sleep apnea. This aspect prohibits the use of portable monitoring as a screening tool to exclude sleep apneas, such as in professional drivers and individuals with supervision tasks (in which symptoms and complaints have not been assessed and may conflict with employability or other issues). Legal issues may become important here as well.

Diagnostic and therapeutic approaches to the management of sleep-disordered breathing differ among countries worldwide.[45] Sleep medicine in some countries is well established, and a significant clinical infrastructure exists. In other countries, economically affordable strategies constitute the primary consideration.[46] In certain settings, sleep medicine may be very basic, with only home sleep testing available for diagnosing sleep apnea.[45] One potential reason for this restriction to home sleep testing alone is the limited availability of sleep medicine centers owing to unmet needs for qualified experts and funding for polysomnography beds. This is the case in countries in which sleep medicine is a young discipline. A second reason is an economic decision to limit access to polysomnography studies to patients with comorbid illnesses. Patients with sleep apnea and no comorbidities are diagnosed with home sleep testing alone. This applies to countries with enough medical resources and a well-developed sleep medicine infrastructure. With improvements in the knowledge base for sleep disorders and sleep-disordered breathing among general physicians, the individual clinician can decide whether a particular patient should be evaluated for suspected sleep apnea alone or exhibits some comorbidity or has other risk factors. Then the patient can be referred for either home sleep testing or cardiorespiratory polysomnography. This approach would allow economic and thoughtful management of patients with respect to diagnosis and subsequent treatment, as appropriate.[13] In Europe, a debate is ongoing that different levels of sleep medicine service include different levels of medical expertise and correspondingly different levels of equipment complexity. Family physicians may have some basic knowledge about sleep-disordered breathing and already sometimes apply simple tests. A limited number of clinical centers would have clinical expertise, training, research, and other technical know-how as required in specialized sleep centers.[46] Many community-based centers have basic sleep medicine knowledge and home sleep testing with four- to six-channel systems.

The other issue is health economy and patient care. A quantitative threshold regarding sleep apnea severity and assessing risk based on evidence still remains to be established. We do not have evidence of how many apneas, how many hypopneas, what duration of apnea events, how much sleep fragmentation, or what degree of hypoxia causes substantial cardiovascular risk with increased mortality. In view of limited therapeutic adherence to CPAP, how strict should researcher-clinicians be with respect to treatment follow-up studies? As the field of sleep medicine approaches the point at which diagnosis can be made easily with home sleep testing, a need is emerging for new clinical evidence and transparent health economic decisions. They are key for developing strategies for managing sleep apnea.[47]

Patients may be diagnosed and even treated at home based on a home sleep apnea test alone. With the COVID-19 pandemic, this management pathway gained popularity among sleep centers. Surveys during the pandemic showed that patients are hesitant to seek medical help when this requires them to physically go to a physician's office or a sleep medicine center.[48] Home sleep apnea testing devices may be sent to a patient and then returned for interpretation of the recording, and an automatic positive airway pressure (APAP) device may be prescribed and delivered to the patient based on the result. Follow-up studies on optimizing pressure settings and checking adherence to the treatment are then performed using telemedicine modalities like medical clouds or secure video-conferencing.[1] One home sleep testing study showed that the 4-week outcome in sleepiness and CPAP adherence was similar to that for sleep laboratory–based diagnosis and treatment.[49] An important limitation of the study was the short follow-up period.[50] Sleep-disordered breathing is a chronic condition, and long-term adherence with CPAP therapy may decline more at home. Thus more research is needed.

Conclusions

Attended clinical polysomnography is the reference standard for diagnosing disordered breathing during sleep. Evidence-based literature, however, indicates that diagnosis of obstructive sleep apnea can be performed using home sleep testing under certain conditions in adults. The recording must include oxygen saturation, airflow, respiratory effort, heart or pulse rate, and body position. The SCOPER parameters summarize these requirements in a comprehensive and quantitative scheme.[5] Visual evaluation is needed to avoid misclassification of sleep apnea severity.[17] It is not possible to distinguish between central and obstructive respiratory events with certainty. Home sleep testing is reliable if it is performed under the supervision of personnel trained in sleep medicine and if screening has been adequate to achieve a high pretest probability among the study subjects suffering from sleep-disordered breathing. In addition, patients should not have other significant sleep or comorbid disorders (e.g., heart failure, stroke, diabetes mellitus, obstructive or restrictive lung diseases, or severe cardiac arrhythmias).

Home sleep testing systems with fewer channels can indicate the likelihood of sleep-disordered breathing but currently are not sufficiently validated for diagnostic purposes. Technological advances are expected to improve these systems. Accordingly, systems with fewer channels may provide a sufficiently reliable diagnosis for disordered breathing during sleep in the near future. High-quality clinical studies with sufficient sample size and comparison against a reference standard are needed.

Technological advances must be accompanied by economy-driven strategies to diagnose and treat patients with sleep apnea.[47] Recent approaches to diagnosing and even treating patients at home seem to provide effectiveness, in terms of outcome, similar to that for sleep laboratory–based studies. Economically proven home-based studies may be more feasible than sleep laboratory–based studies in light of the high prevalence of the disorders and the still-unmet clinical need to recognize and treat patients with sleep-disordered breathing.

Acknowledgments/Disclosures

Several companies have furnished equipment for research or otherwise supported the work on which this chapter is based: Zoll (formerly Itamar Medical, Caesarea, Israel) provided sensors/consumables for research with the Watch-PAT device. Cidelec (Sainte-Gemmes-sur-Loire, France) provided a grant for a validation study of its Pneavox system for laryngeal pressure and sound recording. SleepImage provided their finger ring for evaluating cardiopulmonary coupling in clinical trials. Neurovirtual provided their PSG system for clinical trials. Nox Medical (Reykjavik, Iceland) provided equipment and sensors for testing as part of the European Union Grant no. 965417 "Sleeprevolution." Studies were done at the Interdisciplinary Sleep Medicine Center at Charite-Universitätsmedizin Berlin.

Selected Readings

1. Aurora RN, Swartz R, Punjabi NM. Misclassification of OSA severity with automated scoring of home sleep recordings. *Chest*. 2015;147:719-727.
2. Troester MM, Quan SF, Berry RB, et al. *The AASM Manual for the Scoring of Sleep and Associated Events: Rules, Terminology and Technical Specifications, Version 3*. Darien, IL: American Academy of Sleep Medicine; 2023.
3. Collop N. Home sleep testing: appropriate screening is the key. *Sleep*. 2012;35:1445-1446.
4. El Shayeb M, Topfer LA, Stafinski T, et al. Diagnostic accuracy of level 3 portable sleep tests versus level 1 polysomnography for sleep-disordered breathing: a systematic review and meta-analysis. *CMAJ*. 2014; 186:E25-E51.
5. Kuna ST, Badr MS, Kimoff RJ, et al. An official ATS/AASM/ACCP/ERS Workshop report: research priorities in ambulatory management of adults with obstructive sleep apnea. *Proc Am Thorac Soc*. 2011;8:1-16.
6. Pereira EJ, Driver HS, Stewart SC, Fitzpatrick MF. Comparing a combination of validated questionnaires and level III portable monitor with polysomnography to diagnose and exclude sleep apnea. *J Clin Sleep Med*. 2013;9:1259-1266.
7. Kapur VK, Auckley DH, Chowdhuri S, et al. Clinical practice guideline for diagnostic testing for adult obstructive sleep apnea: an American Academy of Sleep Medicine Clinical Practice Guideline. *J Clin Sleep Med*. 2017;13:479-504.
8. Feltner C, Wallace IF, Aymes S, et al. Screening for obstructive sleep apnea in adults updated evidence report and systematic review for the US Preventive Services Task Force. *JAMA*. 2022;328(19):1951-1971.

References

1. Sico JS, Koo BB, Perkins AJ, et al. Impact of coronavirus disease-2019 pandemic on Veterans Health Administration Sleep Services. *Sage Open Med*. 2023;11:20503121231169388.
2. Collop NA, Anderson WM, Boehlecke B, et al. Clinical guidelines for the use of unattended portable monitors in the diagnosis of obstructive sleep apnea in adult patients. *J Clin Sleep Med*. 2007;3:737-747.
3. Collop NA. Portable monitoring for the diagnosis of obstructive sleep apnea. *Curr Opin Pulm Med*. 2008;14:525-529.
4. Kapur VK, Auckley DH, Chowdhuri S, et al. Clinical practice guideline for diagnostic testing for adult obstructive sleep apnea: an American Academy of Sleep Medicine Clinical Practice Guideline. *J Clin Sleep Med*. 2017;13:479-504.
5. Collop NA, Tracy SL, Kapur V, et al. Obstructive sleep apnea devices for out-of-center (OOC) testing: technology evaluation. *J Clin Sleep Med*. 2011;7:531-548.
6. Kuna ST, Badr MS, Kimoff RJ, et al. An official ATS/AASM/ACCP/ERS workshop report: research priorities in ambulatory management of adults with obstructive sleep apnea. *Proc Am Thorac Soc*. 2011;8: 1-16.
7. Qaseem A, Dallas P, Owens DK, et al. Diagnosis of obstructive sleep apnea in adults: a clinical practice guideline from the American College of Physicians. *Ann Intern Med*. 2014;161:210-220.
8. Penzel T, Blau A, Garcia C, et al. Portable monitoring in sleep apnea. *Curr Respir Care Rep*. 2012;1:139-145.
9. Chesson AL, Berry RB, Pack A. Practice parameters for the use of portable monitoring devices in the investigation of suspected obstructive sleep apnea in adults. *Sleep*. 2003;26:907-913.
10. Flemons WW, Littner MR, Rowley JA, et al. Home diagnosis of sleep apnea: a systematic review of the literature. An evidence review cosponsored by the American Academy of Sleep Medicine, the American College of Chest Physicians, and the American Thoracic Society. *Chest*. 2003;124:1543-1579.
11. Mayer G, Arzt M, Braumann B, et al. German S3 guideline nonrestorative sleep/sleep disorders, chapter sleep-related breathing disorders in adults, short version. *Somnologie (Berl)*. 2017;21:290-230.
12. Pereira EJ, Driver HS, Stwart SC, Fitzpatrick MF. Comparing a combination of validated questionnaires and level III portable monitor with polysomnography to diagnose and exclude sleep apnea. *J Clin Sleep Med*. 2013;9:1259-1266.
13. Feltner C, Wallace IF, Aymes S, et al. Screening for obstructive sleep apnea in adults updated evidence report and systematic review for the US Preventive Services Task Force. *JAMA*. 2022;328(19):1951-1971.
14. Walter J, Lee JY, Blake S, et al. A new wearable diagnostic home sleep testing platform: comparison with available systems and benefits of multinight assessments. *J Clin Sleep Med*. 2023;19:865-872.

15. Practice parameters for the use of portable recording in the assessment of obstructive sleep apnea. Standards of Practice Committee of the American Sleep Disorders Association. *Sleep.* 1994;17:372-377.
16. ATS/ACCP/AASM Taskforce Steering Committee. Executive summary on the systematic review and practice parameters for portable monitoring in the investigation of suspected sleep apnea in adults. *Am J Respir Crit Care Med.* 2004;169:1160-1163.
17. Aurora RN, Swartz R, Punjabi NM. Misclassification of OSA severity with automated scoring of home sleep recordings. *Chest.* 2015;147:719-727.
18. Troester MM, Quan SF, Berry RB, et al. *The AASM Manual for the Scoring of Sleep and Associated Events: Rules, Terminology and Technical Specifications, Version 3.* Darien, IL: American Academy of Sleep Medicine; 2023.
19. Ragette R, Wang Y, Weinreich G, Teschler H. Diagnostic performance of single airflow channel recording (ApneaLink) in home diagnosis of sleep apnea. *Sleep Breath.* 2010;14:109-114.
20. Oktay B, Rice TB, Atwood CW, et al. Evaluation of a single-channel portable monitor for the diagnosis of obstructive sleep apnea. *J Clin Sleep Med.* 2011;7:384-390.
21. Kaniusas E, Pfützner H, Saletu B. Acoustical signal properties for cardiac/respiratory activity and apneas. *IEEE Trans Biomed Eng.* 2005;52:1812-1822.
22. Glos M, Sabil A, Jelavic KS, et al. Characterization of respiratory events in obstructive sleep apnea using suprasternal pressure monitoring. *J Clin Sleep Med.* 2018;14:359-369.
23. Yadollahi A, Giannouli E, Moussavi Z. Sleep apnea monitoring and diagnosis based on pulse oximetry and tracheal sound signals. *Med Biol Eng Comput.* 2010;48:1087-1097.
24. Senny F, Destine J, Poirrier R. Midsagittal jaw movement analysis for the scoring of sleep apneas and hypopneas. *IEEE Trans Biomed Eng.* 2008;55:87-95.
25. Cheliout-Heraut F, Senny F, Djouadi F, et al. Obstructive sleep apnoea syndrome: comparison between polysomnography and portable sleep monitoring based on jaw recordings. *Neurophysiol Clin.* 2011;41:191-198.
26. Senny F, Maury G, Cambron L, et al. The sleep/wake state scoring from mandible movement signal. *Sleep Breath.* 2012;16:535-542.
27. Kelly JL, Ben Messaoud R, Joyeux-Faure M, et al. Diagnosis of sleep apnoea using a mandibular monitor and machine learning analysis: one-night agreement compared to in-home polysomnography. *Front Neurosci.* 2022;16:726880.
28. Bar A, Pillar G, Dvir I, et al. Evaluation of a portable device based on peripheral arterial tone for unattended home sleep studies. *Chest.* 2003;123:695-703.
29. Sommermeyer D, Zou D, Ficker JH, et al. Detection of cardiovascular risk from a photoplethysmographic signal using a matching pursuit algorithm. *Med Biol Eng Comput.* 2016;54:1111-1121.
30. Schnall RP, Sheffy J, Penzel T. Peripheral arterial tonometry—PAT technology. *Sleep Med Rev.* 2022;61:101566.
31. Dvir I, Adler Y, Freiark D, Lavie P. Evidence for fractal correlation properties in variations of peripheral arterial tone during REM sleep. *Am J Physiol Heart Circ Physiol.* 2002;283:H434-H439.
32. De Chazal P, Heneghan C, McNicholas WT. Multimodal detection of sleep apnoea using electrocardiogram and oximetry signals. *Philos Trans A Math Phys Eng Sci.* 2009;367:369-389.
33. Penzel T, Kesper K, Pinnow I, et al. Peripheral arterial tonometry, oximetry and actigraphy for ambulatory recording of sleep apnea. *Physiol Meas.* 2004;25:1025-1036.
34. Yalamanchali S, Farajian V, Hamilton C, et al. Diagnosis of obstructive sleep apnea by peripheral arterial tonometry: meta-analysis. *JAMA Otolaryngol Head Neck Surg.* 2013;139:1343-1350.
35. Guilleminault C, Connolly S, Winkle R, et al. Cyclical variation of the heart rate in sleep apnoea syndrome. Mechanisms, and usefulness of 24 h electrocardiography as a screening technique. *Lancet.* 1984;8369:126-131.
36. Somers VK, Dyken ME, Clary MP, Abboud FM. Sympathetic neural mechanisms in obstructive sleep apnea. *J Clin Invest.* 1995;96:1897-1904.
37. Heneghan C, de Chazal P, Ryan S, et al. Electrocardiogram recording as a screening tool for sleep disordered breathing. *J Clin Sleep Med.* 2008;4:223-228.
38. Mendez MO, Bianchi AM, Mattteucci M, et al. Sleep apnea screening by autoregressive models from a single ECG lead. *IEEE Trans Biomed Eng.* 2009;56:2838-2850.
39. Moody GB, Mark RG, Zoccola A, Mantero S. Clinical validation of the ECG-derived respiration (EDR) technique. *Comput Cardiol.* 1986;13:507-510.

40. Penzel T, McNames J, de Chazal P, et al. Systematic comparison of different algorithms for apnoea detection based on electrocardiogram recordings. *Med Biol Eng Comput*. 2002;40:402-407.
41. Penzel T, Kantelhardt JW, Bartsch RP, et al. Modulations of heart rate, ECG, and cardio-respiratory coupling observed in polysomnography. *Front Physiol*. 2016;7:460.
42. Heneghan C, Chua CP, Garvey JF, et al. A portable automated assessment tool for sleep apnea using a combined Holter-oximeter. *Sleep*. 2008;31:1432-1439.
43. Zamarron C, Gude F, Barcala J, et al. Utility of oxygen saturation and heart rate spectral analysis obtained from pulse oximetric recordings in the diagnosis of sleep apnea syndrome. *Chest*. 2003;123:1567-1576.
44. Raymond B, Cayton RM, Chappell MJ. Combined index of heart rate variability and oximetry in screening for the sleep apnoea/hypopnoea syndrome. *J Sleep Res*. 2003;12:53-61.
45. Fietze I, Laharnar N, Bargiotas P, et al. Management of obstructive sleep apnea in Europe—A 10-year follow-up. *Sleep Med*. 2022;97:64-72.
46. Penzel T, Fietze I, Hirshkowitz M. [Diagnostic pathways in sleep medicine. From a sleep laboratory towards a sleep medicine service structure]. *Somnologie*. 2011;15:78-83.
47. Pevernagie DA, Gnidovec-Strazisar B, Grote L, et al. On the rise and fall of the apnea-hypopnea index: a historical review and critical appraisal. *J Sleep Res*. 2020;29:e13066.
48. Partinen M, Bjorvatn B, Holzinger B, et al. Sleep and circadian problems during the coronavirus disease 2019 (COVID-19) pandemic: the International COVID-19 Sleep Study (ICOSS). *J Sleep Res*. 2021;30(1):e13206.
49. Skomro RP, Gjevre J, Reid J, et al. Outcomes of home-based diagnosis and treatment of obstructive sleep apnea. *Chest*. 2010;138:257-263.
50. Kimoff RJ. To treat or not to treat: can a portable monitor reliably guide decision-making in sleep apnea? *Am J Respir Crit Care Med*. 2011;184:871-872.

CHAPTER 18

Remote Monitoring of Sleep Apnea Patients

Kullatham Kongpakpaisarn ▪ Sritika Thapa ▪ Christine Won

Remote Monitoring of Sleep Apnea Patients

INTRODUCTION TO MODEL OF ASYNCHRONOUS CARE OF SLEEP APNEA PATIENTS

Currently, it is well known that positive airway pressure (PAP) therapy is the first-line and most effective treatment for obstructive sleep apnea (OSA).[1-3] To ensure the proper adherence and optimal therapeutic effect of PAP device, various data management techniques are integrated into current versions of PAP devices so the data can be reviewed by providers and patients. Most PAP devices have built-in data storage that can display basic information through their screen (Figure 18.1) such as total hours of usage, days of usage, mask-fitting quality, and residual apnea-hypopnea index (AHI). If a PAP device is equipped with an SD memory card (Figure 18.2), the data can also be pulled from the card for review. From past to present, sleep medicine practices have recommended that patients bring in their SD memory card for their follow-up visit to ensure treatment efficiency and adherence. Modern PAP devices have built-in modems that can connect directly to the Internet via a cloud system that provides remote monitoring of sleep data on a nightly basis instead of the periodic follow-ups using an SD memory card. Most PAP manufacturers offer computer software or web-based or mobile phone apps (Figure 18.3) that allow patients to access the data for reassurance, engagement, and more informed interaction with their providers.[4] Other sophisticated applications are available and may incur a monthly payment.

Remote monitoring of PAP usage is widely used as it allows disease progression to be followed and new acute events to be detected. Aside from disease monitoring, certain insurance payers, such as Medicare in the United States, requires a face-to-face follow-up visit within 90 days to ensure PAP adherence before authorizing PAP-related supplies.[5] It is currently unclear that remote monitoring itself improves PAP adherence but when combined with telemedicine and certain interventions (e.g., call-based), it is shown to increase minutes per night of PAP usage and the number of patients with ≥4 hours/night adherence.[4]

Continuous Positive Airway Pressure Algorithm for Detecting Respiratory Events

Although there are no available data to confirm the superiority of auto-titrating continuous positive airway pressure (CPAP) devices over manual CPAP and bilevel-positive airway pressure (BIPAP) devices, it is still often preferred in practice to treat sleep apnea.[6-9] In general, auto-titrating CPAP increases airway pressure throughout the inspiratory and expiratory phase and pneumatically stents the airways to prevent collapse during inspiration, thus protecting the

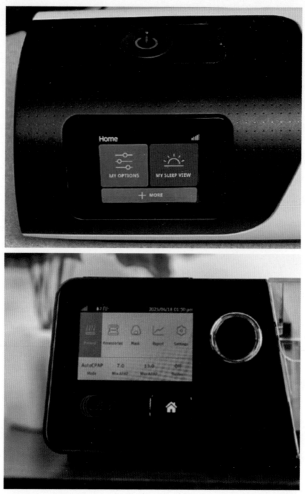

Figure 18.1 PAP machine screen display of patient usage or setting information. *PAP,* Positive airway pressure.

patient from having sleep apnea. Moreover, positive end-expiratory pressure (PEEP) can result in alveoli recruitment, thus further improving ventilation.[10,11]

The main component of an auto-titrating CPAP device consists of sensors, a microprocessor, and a flow generator. Device sensors (flow sensor, altitude sensor, and leak estimator) sense airflow, estimate air leak in the system, and then communicate this information to the microprocessor, which calculates the inspiratory and expiratory circuitry and motor speed. The calculated orders are then transmitted to the flow generator to provide a constant positive pressure to the patient's airway.[12]

In order to have a consistent desired pressure delivered at the patient's airway, the flow must be generated to account for several factors including the length and diameter of the tubing and expected leakage at the mask. Hence, the type of mask (e.g., full face, nasal, pillows) must be input into the device to help it estimate the expected leakage from the system and arrive at the most accurate pressure level for the patient.

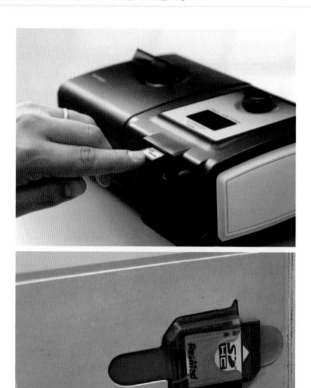

Figure 18.2 SD memory card for a ResMed device.

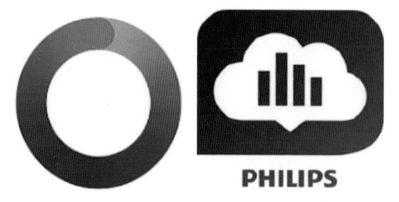

Figure 18.3 MyAir and DreamMapper applications for ResMed and Philips Respironics devices monitoring for patients, respectively.

Each auto-titrating CPAP manufacturer uses a different algorithm to detect apneas and hypopneas, to process the flow signal, and to adjust the amount of positive pressure that is given to the patient. The flow is sampled numerous times throughout 1 second. Artifacts (cough, airway, or cardiac) are removed with a signal filter, and mean flow is determined for a given period. ResMed (ResMed Inc., San Diego, CA) CPAP devices use a breathing index that is calculated from the root mean square (RMS) formula, whereas Philips Respironics devices use a weighted peak flow (WPF) method to estimate the average flow. Other devices such as Lowenstein Prisma APAP or Luna also have their own algorithm to average out the airflow over a given time.

Once the calculated average flow is determined, the device evaluates the data to determine sleep-disordered breathing events. Different devices have different ways for this evaluation. For example, ResMed devices use a 2-second RMS moving average to compare with the prior 1-minute RMS moving average. Philips Respironics devices use a WPF of 1 breath to compare with the mean value of the 80th to 90th percentile of WPFs during the prior 4-minute's moving average.

After flow evaluation, the device then determines sleep-disordered breathing events (apnea or hypopnea) using their proprietary criteria. Table 18.1 summarizes apnea and hypopnea definition for the ResMed AutoSet and Philips Respironics AutoCPAP devices.

Aside from apnea, hypopnea, and flow limitation detection, most devices can also detect vibratory snoring. The response algorithm is unique depending on the device maker and model.

Once upper airway flow limitation, vibratory snoring, or sleep-disordered breathing events (in the absence of central apnea) have been detected, the devices use their algorithm to increase the PAP level until flow or resistance has normalized. Once a therapeutic pressure has been achieved, PAP is reduced until flow limitation or airway resistance normalizes. The pressure-adjusting algorithm on each device is slightly different. ResMed devices increase the pressure level by 3 cmH$_2$O for every 10 seconds of apneic event and 0.6 cmH$_2$O per breath for flow limitation. Philips Respironics devices increase the pressure level by 1 cmH$_2$O over 15 seconds in response to two apneic or hypopneic events or snoring and by 0.5 cmH$_2$O per minute if flow limitation is detected. Thus the time of response varies depending on the CPAP manufacturer or model. Fasquel et al. studied the response time to apnea and hypopnea events by different PAP devices.[13] There is great variability in the amount of pressure and the rate of change in response to obstructive events as well as leakage, depending on the PAP machine model. This should be considered when interpreting the patient's downloaded median and maximum pressure data and when considering narrowing the pressure range. This may also be relevant information when the patient is struggling to acclimate to pressures from their machines. A patient may find that the machine's

TABLE 18.1 ■ Definition of Apnea and Hypopnea for ResMed AutoSet and Phillips Respironics AutoCPAP Devices

Device	Apnea Detection	Hypopnea Detection
ResMed AutoSet	Decreased 2 seconds of RMS moving average of more than 75% from baseline for 10 seconds	Decreased 12 seconds of RMS scaling between 25% and 50% from baseline for 10 seconds with at least 1 obstructed breath in the middle of event
Philips Respironics AutoCPAP	Decreased WPF per breath of more than 80% from baseline for 10 seconds terminating with increased WPF of more than 30% at the end of event (recovery breath)	Decreased WPF per breath between 20% and 60% from baseline for 10 seconds terminating at 60 seconds or with recovery breath over 75% of recent WPF

CPAP, Continuous positive airway pressure; RMS, root mean square; WPF, weighted peak flow.

pressure changes too aggressively, and a general understanding of the different algorithms may help the practitioner determine pressure ranges that improve the patient's experience on their specific PAP machine.

ResMed devices differentiate central from obstructive apnea by using the forced oscillation technique (FOT).[12] The device transmits small oscillation signals into its airflow and detects the bounce-back oscillation. In a closed airway, the oscillation signal reverberates back, which is detected by the device sensor. This apneic event is categorized as obstructive. In an open airway, the oscillation signal dissipates, in which case the event is categorized as central. Philips Respironics devices generate test pressure pulses during apneic events to see if these test pulses can produce airflow. If so, the event is scored as central apnea. Although these techniques are able to detect central apneas, currently there is no PAP device that reliably distinguishes obstructive from central hypopneas. Moreover, the auto-titrating PAP algorithm does not respond to clear airway (central events). Therapeutic pressure will remain the same even after the events are detected. This may warrant a provider to consider a different mode of therapy if excessive central apneas are detected on their device.

Auto-titrating CPAP devices aim to deliver the lowest effective pressure to maintain airway patency. For example, once a normal breathing pattern is achieved, the ResMed device will start gradually decreasing its pressure starting 40 minutes after its last detected apneic event and 20 minutes after the last flow limitation. Philip Respironics devices have a testing protocol before decreasing the pressure. The protocol searches for the critical closing pressure (Pcrit) by ramping down the airway pressure by 0.5 cmH_2O until flow limitation is detected. When detected, the device then automatically increases airway pressure by 1.5 cmH_2O and holds for 10 minutes. After stable breathing is restored, the device then ramps up airway pressure by 0.5 cmH_2O again. If there is no further improvement in the airflow, the device then decreases the pressure down by 1.5 cmH_2O, and settles on this as its optimal pressure (Popt).[12]

Using Downloads to Optimize Care

It is recommended that patients with sleep apnea follow with their providers every 6 to 12 months. At each visit, CPAP data download would be assessed to optimize sleep apnea treatment. The data download is different for each manufacturer but generally consists of date of pulled data, adherence report (average time of usage), model, settings, and therapeutic reports (pressure, leak, and residual events). See Figures 18.4 and 18.5.

Usage (Adherence Report)

Most insurance payers follow Centers for Medicare and Medicaid Services (CMS) guidelines and define *PAP adherence* as using the device for therapy (1) more than 4 hours per night and (2) at least 70% of the nights during any consecutive 30-day period during the first 3 months of usage.[5] *PAP non-adherence* is defined as usage that does not meet the CMS guideline, and it is very common among PAP users.[14,15] Multiple factors are associated with PAP non-adherence.[16] Some of the factors such as demographics (age, gender, ethnicity, socioeconomic status) or disease severity and symptoms are not likely to be easily modified. On the other hand, side effects of PAP therapy (e.g., xerostomia, nasal congestion, aerophagia, mask leak) could be accessed by patients' history taking combined with a PAP data report and subsequently addressed to improve adherence. Telemedicine has been used to improve PAP adherence, although the effectiveness is still unclear.[16] Hwang et al. found that CPAP telemonitoring with automated feedback improved 90-day CPAP adherence in OSA patients, but telemedicine-based education showed no significant improvement in PAP adherence.[17]

Positive Airway Pressure Mode

Modes for PAP therapy include CPAP, BPAP, adaptive servoventilation (ASV), and volume-assured pressure support (VAPS). CPAP, which is the most commonly used mode, provides a continuous pressure level throughout the therapeutic period. BPAP provides two levels of pressure during inspiration (IPAP) and expiration (EPAP). ASV is primarily used to treat central sleep apnea.[18] It provides two pressure levels like BPAP, with an additional function to adjust the pressure delivery using an integrative sensor that detects respiratory airflow with a set backup rate.

Usage				03/07/2022 - 04/05/2022
Usage days				30/30 days (100%)
>= 4 hours				30 days (100%)
< 4 hours				0 days (0%)
Usage hours				248 hours 7 minutes
Average usage (total days)				8 hours 16 minutes
Average usage (days used)				8 hours 16 minutes
Median usage (days used)				8 hours 9 minutes
Total used hours (value since last reset - 04/05/2022)				14,535 hours

AirSense 10 AutoSet	
Serial number	
Mode	AutoSet
Min Pressure	6 cmH2O
Max Pressure	12 cmH2O
EPR	Fulltime
EPR level	2
Response	Standard

Therapy						
Pressure - cmH2O	Median:	6.9	95th percentile:	8.7	Maximum:	10.0
Leaks - L/min	Median:	0.0	95th percentile:	5.7	Maximum:	15.6
Events per hour	AI:	0.8	HI:	0.1	AHI:	0.9
Apnea Index	Central:	0.0	Obstructive:	0.8	Unknown:	0.0
RERA Index						0.0
Cheyne-Stokes respiration (average duration per night)						0 minutes (0%)

Usage - hours

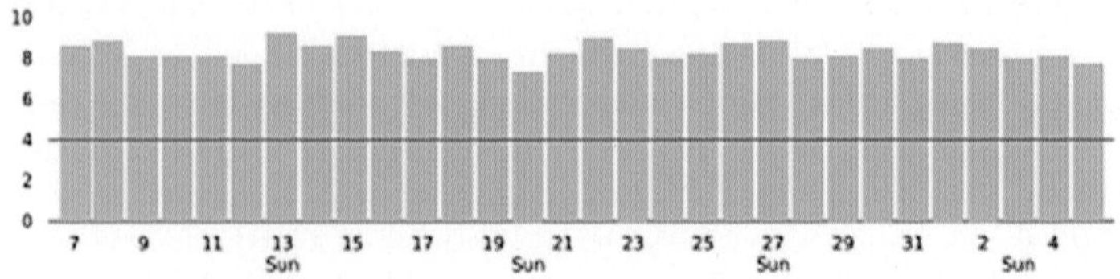

Figure 18.4 Data download from ResMed device.

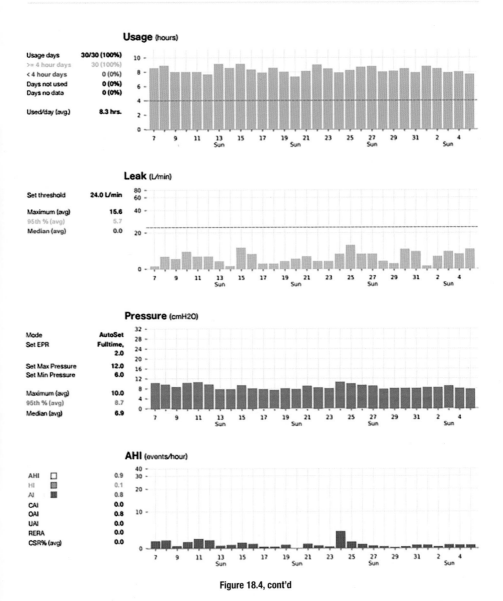

Figure 18.4, cont'd

VAPS automatically adjusts pressure support levels to match a set tidal volume or alveolar ventilation to guarantee adequate ventilation.

Therapeutic Pressure Values

Pressure values that are commonly reported in PAP data download include mean/median pressure, 90th or 95th percentile pressure, and maximal/peak pressure. Mean/median pressure is the average pressure level that the PAP device provides from the start to the end of therapy, whereas 90th or 95th percentile pressure is considered as the most effective pressure for the patient.

It means that the patient has spent 90% or 95% of their PAP therapy at or below this pressure level, respectively. Maximal/peak pressure is the highest amount of pressure that the PAP device reached throughout the therapeutic period. The most common empiric pressure setting for auto-titrating CPAP is 4 to 20 cmH$_2$O. Unfortunately, this can lead to suboptimal treatment, especially in patients with supine- or REM-predominant sleep apnea, who typically have higher pressure requirements during supine position or REM sleep than their baseline. Based on current algorithms for pressure delivery, most devices are unable to increase the pressure adequately over a short period to sufficiently overcome flow limitation during REM or supine sleep, often leaving patients with high residual respiratory events and marked desaturations. Thus most experts recommend narrowing PAP ranges once the patient's optimal pressure is determined.

Respiratory Events

The events are reported in the form of average AHI throughout the hours of usage. Each PAP model has its own unique algorithm to determine the respiratory events as mentioned in the previous section. Most PAP devices can distinguish between obstructive apnea and hypopnea events, but currently there are no devices that can reliably detect central hypopneas. One study compared the accuracy of a PAP device to a titration polysomnography for detecting AHI and found a high correlation for residual obstructive AHI, but a low correlation for central AHI.[19]

In ResMed devices, "unknown apneas" are reported. In the ResMed S8 and prior models, unknown events suggest any type of apnea that occurs at PAP levels above 10 cmH$_2$O. However, in S9 to current models, unknown apneas indicate events that are associated with high leakage over 30 L/min. In these cases, apneas may be occurring due to ineffective pressure delivery from high leaks, or because high leaks impair the machine from accurately categorizing an apnea.

Respiratory effort–related arousals (RERAs) are a milder form of respiratory disturbance consisting of increased airway resistance associated with arousals and sleep disturbance. RERAs

Compliance Information   9/15/2023 - 10/14/2023   **A-Flex™**

Compliance Summary

Date Range	9/15/2023 - 10/14/2023 (30 days)
Days with Device Usage	30 days
Days without Device Usage	0 days
Percent Days with Device Usage	100.0%
Cumulative Usage	8 days 18 hrs. 11 mins. 44 secs.
Maximum Usage (1 Day)	8 hrs. 29 mins. 19 secs.
Average Usage (All Days)	7 hrs. 23 secs.
Average Usage (Days Used)	7 hrs. 23 secs.
Minimum Usage (1 Day)	5 hrs. 5 mins. 34 secs.
Percent of Days with Usage >= 4 Hours	100.0%
Percent of Days with Usage < 4 Hours	0.0%
Total Blower Time	8 days 20 hrs. 23 mins. 22 secs.

Auto-CPAP Summary (Philips Respironics)

Auto-CPAP Mean Pressure	8.3 cmH2O
Auto-CPAP Peak Average Pressure	10.8 cmH2O
Device Pressure <= 90% of Time	9.0 cmH2O
Average Time in Large Leak Per Day	2 mins. 28 secs.
Average AHI	2.0

Figure 18.5   Data download from Philips Respironics device.

Device Settings as of	10/14/2023
Device Mode	AutoCPAP - A-Flex

Device Settings

Parameter	Value
Min Pressure	8 cmH2O
Max Pressure	20 cmH2O
A-Flex Setting	1
Auto Off	Off
Auto On	On
View Optional Screens	On
Ramp	Off
Mask Alert	Off
Mask Resistance	2
Mask Resistance Lock	Off
Tubing Type	22
Tubing Type Lock	Off
Opti-Start	Off
Mask Reminder Period	Off
Change Humidifier Settings	Yes
Humidification Mode	Classic
Humidifier Setting	Off
Instant Message Text	

Figure 18.5, cont'd

are commonly reported metrics on PAP devices. However, RERAs as measured by a PAP machine are inherently different than RERAs diagnosed by polysomnography because the PAP machine has no way of measuring sleep and wake states. On a PAP machine, it is defined as a sequence of breaths with small reductions in airflow during a 10-second period that terminates with a sudden increase in airflow.

Leaks

There are two types of leakage from PAP usage: expected leak and unintentional leak. Unintentional leak is the most frequently reported side effect of PAP therapy and generally results from poor mask fit or seal. Less frequently, there may be high unintentional leaks resulting from poor integrity of the hose or connections. For ResMed devices, leaks are reported in liters per minute (L/min) during mean, 95th percentile, and maximal pressures, whereas Respironics devices report the amount of time with large leak (>50–70 L/min). In general, a leak rate should be less than 24 L/min (i.e., expected leak) for ResMed devices. For Respironics devices, time of large leak that is less than 1 hour is generally considered acceptable or non-problematic.[20] High air leak should be addressed because it is associated with poor adherence, sleep interruption, patient discomfort, and affects the efficacy of PAP therapy. When there is a high leak, the auto-titrating PAP increases its pressure delivery to compensate, which could lead to further leak and patient discomfort. Therefore when addressing a high residual AHI related to high leaks, the leaks should be addressed before adjusting PAP settings.

Comfort Setting

More than one-half of patients on PAP therapy experience side effects (i.e., xerostomia, aerosuffocation, or air leak) that lead to sleep interruption during PAP therapy and thus reduce overall adherence.[14] Comfort modes are features that are optional and may be used to improve the patient's sleep experience.

ResMed PAP devices have an *Expiratory Pressure Relief (EPR)* feature that drops the pressure at the start of expiration to allow for less resistance during exhalation. The drop in expiratory pressure is sustained throughout the expiration period. It can be set from 0 to 3 cmH$_2$O. Philips Respironics devices have a *C-Flex* feature that functions similarly but only drops the pressure at the beginning of the exhalation period. *A-Flex* is very similar to *C-Flex* in terms of functionality, but it can provide a smooth pressure increment during the inhalation period as well.

Certain devices take into consideration different OSA phenotypes. For example, females tend to have a lower arousal threshold during non-rapid eye movement (NREM) sleep[21] and therefore may be more likely to awaken and have their sleep disrupted by rapid pressure changes. ResMed designed a machine called ResMed AutoSet for Her that is specific to this issue by creating a female-specific algorithm with slower pressure changes aimed at preventing sleep disturbances in high-arousal threshold PAP users (Table 18.2). McArdle et al. compared ResMed AutoSet for

TABLE 18.2 ■ Comparing Algorithm Between ResMed AutoSet and ResMed AutoSet for Her

Device	PAP Response to Obstructive Events (Apnea and Hypopnea)	PAP Response to Flow Limitation and Vibratory Snoring	PAP Decrement Protocol
ResMed AutoSet	Maximum increment of 3 cmH$_2$O in 10 seconds	Maximum increment of 0.6 cmH$_2$O per breath	PAP gradually decreases 40 minutes after apnea or 20 minutes after flow limitation
ResMed AutoSet for Her	Maximum increment of 2.5 cmH$_2$O in 10 seconds	Maximum increment of 0.5 cmH$_2$O per breath	PAP gradually decreases 40 minutes after apnea, 20 minutes after snoring, and 60 minutes after flow limitation

PAP, Positive airway pressure.

Her with ResMed S9 AutoSet in 20 female patients who were well established on PAP therapy and found no inferiority to S9 AutoSet. However, subjective measurements including comfort of breathing, ease of falling asleep, sleep disturbance, and refreshed feeling were also not significantly different between devices.[22] Newer ResMed devices have an option to choose the intensity of response to flow limitation. For example, *soft response* allows for a gentler pressure response to flow limitation at pressures over 10 cmH$_2$O.

Another function of ResMed's device *climate setting* consists of two components: the humidity and air temperature. The *climate setting* can be set in automatic or manual mode. When set to automatic mode, the humidifier adjusts humidity output based on temperature inside the host to maintain a constant, comfortable humidity level at 85% of relative humidity. In other words, the warmer the temperature of the air, the more humidity output will be added. And the opposite happens for lower temperature. For the tube temperature, when set at automatic mode, the device maintains temperature by adjusting the heated coil inside the tube to aim for 80° Fahrenheit or 27° Celsius. In the manual mode, a patient can choose the level of humidity and tube temperature that is most comfortable to sleep and avoid xerostomia.

Ramp is a feature that helps new PAP users adapt to therapy. It works by starting therapy at a lower pressure instead of therapeutic pressure. If Ramp is set at a fixed ramp, the starting pressure could be as low as 4 or 5 cmH$_2$O and gradually increase over a set period. ResMed devices have an *AutoRamp* function that increases airway pressure only after sleep onset is inferred and then increases the pressure by 1 cmH$_2$O per minute until it reaches target pressure. With this machine, sleep onset is assumed when there are 30 breaths of stable breathing or when three obstructive apneic or hypopneic events are detected within a 2-minute period. If sleep onset is not detected, the machine increases pressure to target level within 30 minutes. Similarly, Philips Respironics devices have a *SmartRamp* function that detects apneic or hypopneic events during the ramp time and adjusts airway pressure when the event is detected. In addition, *EZ-start* is a feature of the newer Philips Respironics CPAP device that increases the starting CPAP level by 1 cmH$_2$O on each successful night (defined as usage of more than 4 hours) until the prescribed pressure is reached (Figure 18.6).

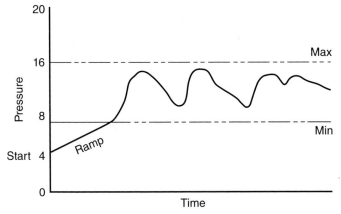

Figure 18.6   ResMed's fixed Ramp.

Case Examples

There are no standard clinical guidelines for how to respond to data downloads during follow-up visits in sleep apnea patients. Each case is unique and requires a thorough clinical evaluation and personal considerations. The following are examples of PAP cases that are typically seen in the sleep medicine clinic.

Usage	01/22/2023 - 02/20/2023
Usage days	30/30 days (100%)
>= 4 hours	30 days (100%)
< 4 hours	0 days (0%)
Usage hours	204 hours 19 minutes
Average usage (total days)	6 hours 49 minutes
Average usage (days used)	6 hours 49 minutes
Median usage (days used)	6 hours 52 minutes
Total used hours (value since last reset - 02/20/2023)	2,141 hours

AirSense 11 AutoSet	
Serial number	22211796104
Mode	AutoSet
Min Pressure	7 cmH2O
Max Pressure	14 cmH2O
EPR	Fulltime
EPR level	2
Response	Standard

Therapy						
Pressure - cmH2O	Median:	8.7	95th percentile:	10.9	Maximum:	11.9
Leaks - L/min	Median:	0.0	95th percentile:	3.7	Maximum:	17.2
Events per hour	AI:	0.1	HI:	0.0	AHI:	0.1
Apnea Index	Central:	0.0	Obstructive:	0.0	Unknown:	0.0
RERA Index						0.0
Cheyne-Stokes respiration (average duration per night)						0 minutes (0%)

Usage - hours

CASE 1

JE is a 58-year-old female patient with moderate OSA who had been established on CPAP therapy. The patient presents to the sleep clinic for her annual follow-up examination. She expresses great benefit from CPAP and feels very comfortable using the device. Her data download demonstrates excellent adherence, low leakage, and low residual AHI. The provider makes no adjustment to her PAP settings. Her PAP supplies are renewed, and she is scheduled to be seen the following year.

Usage	04/26/2023 - 05/25/2023
Usage days	**13/30 days (43%)**
>= 4 hours	**1 days (3%)**
< 4 hours	**12 days (40%)**
Usage hours	33 hours 14 minutes
Average usage (total days)	1 hours 6 minutes
Average usage (days used)	2 hours 33 minutes
Median usage (days used)	2 hours 31 minutes
Total used hours (value since last reset - 05/25/2023)	107 hours

AirSense 11 AutoSet	
Serial number	
Mode	AutoSet
Min Pressure	5 cmH2O
Max Pressure	20 cmH2O
EPR	Fulltime
EPR level	2
Response	Standard

Therapy						
Pressure - cmH2O	Median:	6.4	95th percentile:	8.1	Maximum:	8.8
Leaks - L/min	Median:	0.0	95th percentile:	0.0	Maximum:	2.8
Events per hour	AI:	0.3	HI:	0.3	AHI:	0.6
Apnea Index	Central:	0.1	Obstructive:	0.2	Unknown:	0.0
RERA Index						0.1
Cheyne-Stokes respiration (average duration per night)						0 minutes (0%)

Usage - hours

CASE 2

RC is a 55-year-old female patient who was diagnosed with severe REM-related OSA. She was established on auto-titrating CPAP therapy with a range of 5 to 20 cmH$_2$O. The patient is able to fall asleep quickly with the machine on, but she is awoken abruptly after about 1 to 2 hours gasping with feelings of suffocation and unable to fall back asleep or unintentionally ripping the mask off her face. She ends up sleeping the rest of the night without it. She is brought in for a titration study, where it is noted that she requires only 6 cmH$_2$O to stabilize breathing during NREM sleep, but requires up to 15 cmH$_2$O during supine REM sleep. With these findings, it is now understood why the patient is unable to tolerate the machine for more than 2 hours at a time. It appears that a mean CPAP of 6.4 cmH$_2$O was sufficient to control OSA during NREM sleep, but when the patient entered REM sleep after about 2 hours, the setting was too low to treat her REM-OSA, causing breakthrough events that led to abrupt awakenings and feelings of suffocation. Based on the titration study, the auto-titrating CPAP is adjusted to 13 to 18 cmH_2O to provide the comfort of lower pressures during NREM sleep but high enough to be able to quickly ramp to therapeutic pressures during REM sleep. With these pressure changes, acclimation exercises, and a long ramp time, the patient is eventually able to fall asleep and sleep through the night on PAP therapy.

Compliance Summary

Date Range	3/12/2022 - 4/10/2022 (30 days)
Days with Device Usage	26 days
Days without Device Usage	4 days
Percent Days with Device Usage	86.7%
Cumulative Usage	9 days 1 hrs. 9 mins. 30 secs.
Maximum Usage (1 Day)	9 hrs. 54 mins. 11 secs.
Average Usage (All Days)	7 hrs. 14 mins. 19 secs.
Average Usage (Days Used)	8 hrs. 21 mins. 8 secs.
Minimum Usage (1 Day)	7 hrs. 1 mins. 35 secs.
Percent of Days with Usage >= 4 Hours	86.7%
Percent of Days with Usage < 4 Hours	13.3%
Total Blower Time	9 days 1 hrs. 9 mins. 45 secs.

Auto-CPAP Summary

Auto-CPAP Mean Pressure	8.4 cmH2O
Auto-CPAP Peak Average Pressure	12.0 cmH2O
Device Pressure <= 90% of Time	11.0 cmH2O
Average Time in Large Leak Per Day	6 mins. 14 secs.
Average AHI	7.5

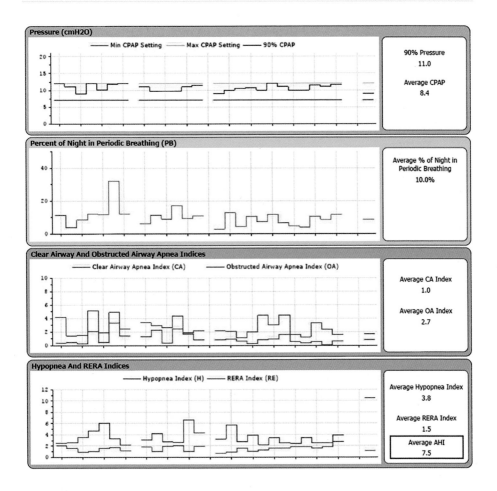

CASE 3

RP is a 66-year-old male patient with moderate OSA and atrial fibrillation. The patient presents to the sleep clinic for a follow-up after 1 year of CPAP therapy. He reports that he is more symptomatic from atrial fibrillation, and his cardiologist is considering catheter ablation. His sleep quality has also worsened recently with more frequent awakenings despite continuing to wear his PAP nightly. Data download demonstrates a slightly increased residual AHI of 7.5 (central apnea index, 1.0; obstructive apnea index, 2.7; hypopnea index, 3.8) with periodic breathing occurring on average 10% of the night. Even though the AHI is only mildly elevated, the patient is symptomatic with poor sleep despite PAP therapy. It is difficult to conclude based on the download alone whether these abnormalities represent Cheyne-Stokes breathing, paroxysmal nocturnal dyspnea, or treatment-emergent central sleep apnea (TE-CSA), all of which are known to occur more frequently with atrial fibrillation,[23] versus residual OSA or falsely detected events. Given the change in symptoms associated with changes in the downloaded data and a broad differential for the elevated AHI and periodic breathing, it is decided to bring the patient in for an in-laboratory titration study.

Compliance Summary

Date Range	1/11/2023 - 2/9/2023 (30 days)
Days with Device Usage	29 days
Days without Device Usage	1 day
Percent Days with Device Usage	96.7%
Cumulative Usage	8 days 6 hrs. 36 mins. 11 secs.
Maximum Usage (1 Day)	11 hrs. 57 mins. 23 secs.
Average Usage (All Days)	6 hrs. 37 mins. 12 secs.
Average Usage (Days Used)	6 hrs. 50 mins. 54 secs.
Minimum Usage (1 Day)	4 hrs. 2 mins. 37 secs.
Percent of Days with Usage >= 4 Hours	96.7%
Percent of Days with Usage < 4 Hours	3.3%
Total Blower Time	8 days 15 hrs. 6 mins. 33 secs.

Auto-CPAP Summary

Auto-CPAP Mean Pressure	11.2 cmH2O
Auto-CPAP Peak Average Pressure	20.0 cmH2O
Device Pressure <= 90% of Time	17.9 cmH2O
Average Time in Large Leak Per Day	4 secs.
Average AHI	14.6

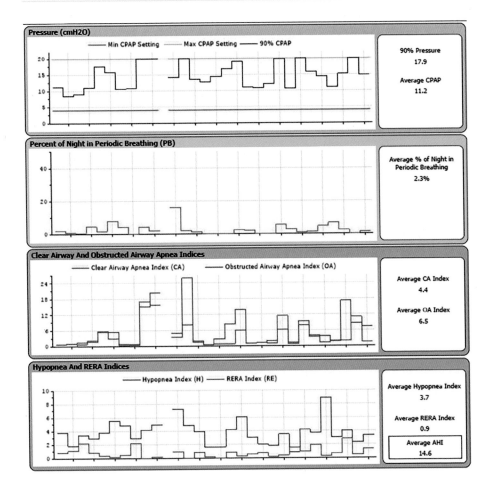

CASE 4

JF is a 67-year-old male patient with severe OSA. The patient presents to the sleep clinic for a semiannual follow-up examination. He expresses persistent daytime sleepiness and fragmented sleep. Data download demonstrates good adherence, low leakage, but high residual AHI. His average 90th percentile pressure over the course of the reported 30 days is 18 cmH$_2$O, and on many nights his 90th percentile pressure reaches the maximum pressure of 20 cmH$_2$O. The patient likely requires a higher PAP setting to treat his severe OSA. He is brought in for an in-laboratory titration study with BPAP therapy in which pressures up to 25 cmH$_2$O may be used while evaluating for emergence of central apneas under these high-pressure settings.

Usage	02/07/2022 - 03/08/2022
Usage days	29/30 days (97%)
>= 4 hours	29 days (97%)
< 4 hours	0 days (0%)
Usage hours	249 hours 42 minutes
Average usage (total days)	8 hours 19 minutes
Average usage (days used)	8 hours 37 minutes
Median usage (days used)	8 hours 39 minutes
Total used hours (value since last reset - 03/08/2022)	376 hours

AirCurve 10 VAuto	
Serial number	23212951489
Mode	Spont
IPAP	16 cmH2O
EPAP	8 cmH2O
Easy-Breathe	On

Therapy						
Leaks – L/min	Median:	0.0	95th percentile:	2.5	Maximum:	8.9
Events per hour	AI:	0.4	HI:	0.1	AHI:	0.5
Apnea Index	Central:	0.0	Obstructive:	0.4	Unknown:	0.0

Usage - hours

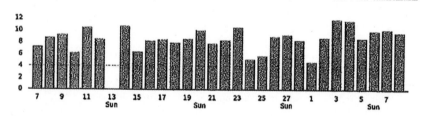

CASE 5

KK is a 69-year-old male patient with severe OSA, chronic obstructive pulmonary disease (COPD), and morbid obesity (body mass index [BMI], 51.4 kg/m^2) who previously failed auto-titrating CPAP due to high residual AHI and unresolved daytime sleepiness. BPAP therapy was prescribed. The patient presents to the sleep clinic for a follow-up visit. His data download demonstrates excellent adherence, low residual AHI, and no leakage. Despite the usage, he reports no improvement in his symptoms of sleepiness and morning headaches. There is concern for persistent sleep-disordered breathing despite a normalized AHI,[24] in the form of sleep-related hypoxemia or hypoventilation. An overnight oximetry on BPAP therapy is ordered.

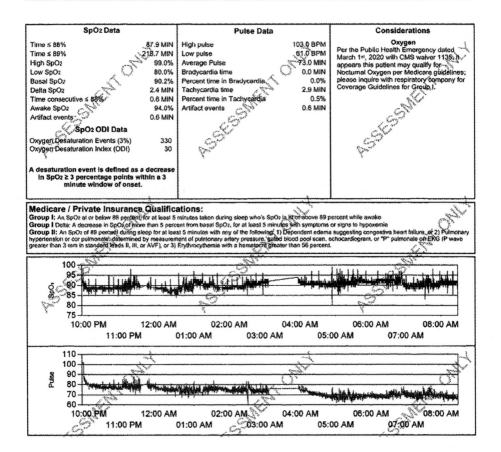

SpO2 Data		Pulse Data		Considerations
Time ≤ 88%	87.9 MIN	High pulse	103.0 BPM	**Oxygen**
Time ≤ 89%	218.7 MIN	Low pulse	61.0 BPM	Per the Public Health Emergency dated March 1st, 2020 with CMS waiver 1135, it appears this patient may qualify for Nocturnal Oxygen per Medicare guidelines; please inquire with respiratory company for Coverage Guidelines for Group I.
High SpO2	99.0%	Average Pulse	73.0 MIN	
Low SpO2	80.0%	Bradycardia time	0.0 MIN	
Basal SpO2	90.2%	Percent time in Bradycardia	0.0%	
Delta SpO2	2.4 MIN	Tachycardia time	2.9 MIN	
Time consecutive ≤ 88%	0.6 MIN	Percent time in Tachycardia	0.5%	
Awake SpO2	94.0%	Artifact events	0.6 MIN	
Artifact events	0.6 MIN			

SpO2 ODI Data

Oxygen Desaturation Events (3%)	330
Oxygen Desaturation Index (ODI)	30

A desaturation event is defined as a decrease in SpO2 ≥ 3 percentage points within a 3 minute window of onset.

Medicare / Private Insurance Qualifications:
Group I: An SpO2 at or below 88 percent, for at least 5 minutes taken during sleep who's SpO2 is at or above 89 percent while awake
Group I Delta: A decrease in SpO2 of more than 5 percent from basal SpO2, for at least 5 minutes with symptoms or signs to hypoxemia
Group II: An SpO2 of 89 percent during sleep for at least 5 minutes with any of the following: 1) Dependent edema suggesting congestive heart failure, or 2) Pulmonary hypertension or cor pulmonale, determined by measurement of pulmonary artery pressure, gated blood pool scan, echocardiogram, or "P" pulmonale on EKG (P wave greater than 3 mm in standard leads II, III, or AVF), or 3) Erythrocythemia with a hematocrit greater than 56 percent.

His overnight oximetry while on BPAP shows an elevated oxygen desaturation index (ODI) of 30 events per hour and mild nocturnal hypoxemia with a mean SpO_2 of 90%, supporting the provider's hypothesis of poorly controlled OSA as well as COPD-related hypoxemia and/or COPD- or obesity-related hypoventilation. The patient is sent for an in-laboratory BPAP titration study with transcutaneous carbon dioxide ($TcCO_2$) monitoring.

Usage	04/24/2023 - 05/23/2023
Usage days	**27/30 days (90%)**
>= 4 hours	**0 days (0%)**
< 4 hours	**27 days (90%)**
Usage hours	18 hours 7 minutes
Average usage (total days)	36 minutes
Average usage (days used)	40 minutes
Median usage (days used)	37 minutes
Total used hours (value since last reset - 05/23/2023)	96 hours

AirSense 11 AutoSet	
Serial number	23221508440
Mode	AutoSet
Min Pressure	5 cmH2O
Max Pressure	20 cmH2O
EPR	Ramp Only
EPR level	1
Response	Standard

Therapy						
Pressure - cmH2O	Median:	4.4	95th percentile:	6.6	Maximum:	7.7
Leaks - L/min	Median:	37.6	95th percentile:	90.4	Maximum:	99.0
Events per hour	AI:	9.0	HI:	0.0	AHI:	9.0
Apnea Index	Central:	0.0	Obstructive:	2.2	Unknown:	6.8
RERA Index						0.0
Cheyne-Stokes respiration (average duration per night)						**0 minutes (0%)**

Usage - hours

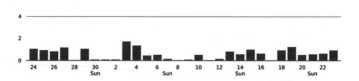

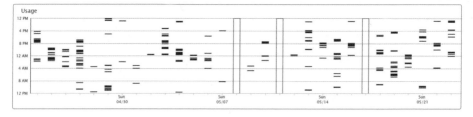

CASE 6

BS is a 70-year-old male patient with severe OSA who was just established on CPAP therapy. The patient presents to the sleep clinic for a 90-day follow-up examination. He reports putting the mask on almost every night and even during the daytime as he tries to acclimate to the machine, however, he is unable to keep the mask on for more than a few minutes at a time. Data download demonstrates his efforts. It also shows high leakage, high residual AHI (predominantly unknown events), and fragmented usage throughout the night (likely due to the automatic start and stop function). Given the low usage time, it is difficult to make any conclusions about the residual AHI and pressure needs. Based on further discussion with the patient, it appears that the patient was wearing his mask incorrectly, leading to large mask leaks and intolerance for extended periods. The patient is scheduled for a mask fitting and education along with a follow-up examination in 6 weeks to assess his progress.

Usage days	29/30 days (97%)
>= 4 hours	23 days (77%)
< 4 hours	6 days (20%)
Usage hours	144 hours 10 minutes
Average usage (total days)	4 hours 48 minutes
Average usage (days used)	4 hours 58 minutes
Median usage (days used)	5 hours 0 minutes
Total used hours (value since last reset - 11/26/2022)	700 hours

AirSense 11 AutoSet

Serial number	22212027938
Mode	AutoSet
Min Pressure	5 cmH2O
Max Pressure	20 cmH2O
EPR	Fulltime
EPR level	3
Response	Standard

Therapy

Pressure - cmH2O	Median:	6.2	95th percentile:	8.3	Maximum:	9.8
Leaks - L/min	Median:	3.4	95th percentile:	19.3	Maximum:	29.3
Events per hour	AI:	8.2	HI:	0.6	AHI:	8.8
Apnea Index	Central:	6.7	Obstructive:	1.1	Unknown:	0.3
RERA Index						0.1

Cheyne-Stokes respiration (average duration per night)	3 minutes (1%)

Usage - hours

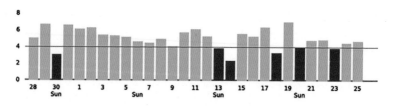

AHI	☐	8.8
HI	▦	0.6
AI	■	8.2
CAI		6.7
OAI		1.1
UAI		0.3
RERA		0.1
CSR% (avg)		1.2

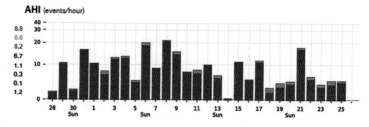

CASE 7

AL is a 77-year-old male patient with mild symptomatic OSA who is newly established on CPAP therapy. Data download demonstrates his usage. The patient does not note any improvement in his sleep symptoms. His residual AHI initially was elevated with a central predominance, raising concerns for TE-CSA. It is noted that his adherence begins to decline after a couple of weeks in the setting of persistently elevated AHI and lack of symptom improvement. Although his usage hours decreased somewhat, his AHI improved in the more recent days. A comparison of days with high AHI to recent days with improved AHI shows marked improvement in leaks. Because high leaks are a risk factor for TE-CSA, it is decided to aggressively control leaks and follow up a download in the next few weeks to ensure resolution of TE-CSA and overall improvement in usage hours.

References

1. Gottlieb DJ, Punjabi NM. Diagnosis and management of obstructive sleep apnea: a review. *JAMA*. 2020;323(14):1389-1400.
2. Gambino F, Zammuto MM, Virzì A, et al. Treatment options in obstructive sleep apnea. *Intern Emerg Med*. 2022;17(4):971-978.
3. Lorenzi-Filho G, Almeida FR, Strollo PJ. Treating OSA: current and emerging therapies beyond CPAP. *Respirology*. 2017;22(8):1500-1507.
4. Labarca G, Schmidt A, Dreyse J, et al. Telemedicine interventions for CPAP adherence in obstructive sleep apnea patients: systematic review and meta-analysis. *Sleep Med Rev*. 2021;60:101543.
5. Centers for Medicare and Medicaid Services. *Decision memo for Continuous Positive Airway Pressure (CPAP) Therapy for Obstructive Sleep Apnea (OSA) (CAG-00093N)*. Available at: https://www.cms.gov/medicare-coverage-database/view/ncacal-decision-memo.aspx?proposed=N&NCAId=19&fromdb=true. Accessed March 1, 2024.
6. Dinh-Thi-Dieu H, Vo-Thi-Kim A, Tran-Van H, Duong-Quy S. Efficacy and adherence of auto-CPAP therapy in patients with obstructive sleep apnea: a prospective study. *Multidiscip Respir Med*. 2020; 15(1):468.
7. Hertegonne K, Bauters F. The value of auto-adjustable CPAP devices in pressure titration and treatment of patients with obstructive sleep apnea syndrome. *Sleep Med Rev*. 2010;14(2):115-119.
8. Lebret M, Rotty MC, Argento C, et al. Comparison of auto- and fixed-continuous positive airway pressure on air leak in patients with obstructive sleep apnea: data from a randomized controlled trial. *Can Respir J*. 2019;2019:6310956.
9. Pływaczewski R, Zgierska A, Bednarek M, Zieliński J. Porównanie automatycznego (AUTO-CPAP) i "ręcznego" doboru ciśnienia leczniczego u chorych na obturacyjny bezdech senny (OBS) [Comparison of automatic (AUTO-CPAP)and "manual" CPAP pressure titration in patients with obstructive sleep apnea]. *Pneumonol Alergol Pol*. 2000;68(5-6):232-237.
10. Berry RB, Parish JM, Hartse KM. The use of auto-titrating continuous positive airway pressure for treatment of adult obstructive sleep apnea. An American Academy of Sleep Medicine review. *Sleep*. 2002;25(2):148-173.
11. Krieger J. Therapeutic use of auto-CPAP. *Sleep Med Rev*. 1999;3(2):159-174.
12. *Advances in the Diagnosis and Treatment of Sleep Apnea: Filling the Gap Between Physicians and Engineers*. Cham: Springer International Publishing; 2022.
13. Fasquel L, Yazdani P, Zaugg C, et al. Impact of unintentional air leaks on automatic positive airway pressure device performance in simulated sleep apnea events. *Respir Care*. 2023;68(1):31-37.
14. Bros J, Poulet C, Methni JE, et al. Determination of risks of lower adherence to CPAP treatment before their first use by patients. *J Health Psychol*. 2022;27(1):223-235.
15. Rotenberg BW, Murariu D, Pang KP. Trends in CPAP adherence over twenty years of data collection: a flattened curve. *J Otolaryngol Head Neck Surg*. 2016;45(1):43.
16. Mehrtash M, Bakker JP, Ayas N. Predictors of continuous positive airway pressure adherence in patients with obstructive sleep apnea. *Lung*. 2019;197(2):115-121.

17. Hwang D, Chang JW, Benjafield AV, et al. Effect of telemedicine education and telemonitoring on continuous positive airway pressure adherence. The Tele-OSA Randomized Trial. *Am J Respir Crit Care Med.* 2018;197(1):117-126.
18. Javaheri S, Brown LK, Randerath WJ. Positive airway pressure therapy with adaptive servoventilation: part 1: operational algorithms. *Chest.* 2014;146(2):514-523.
19. Richter M, Schroeder M, Domanski U, et al. Reliability of respiratory event detection with continuous positive airway pressure in moderate to severe obstructive sleep apnea—comparison of polysomnography with a device-based analysis. *Sleep Breath.* 2023;27(4):1639-1650.
20. OSCAR leaks. Available at: https://www.apneaboard.com/wiki/index.php/OSCAR_leaks#Difference_between_Total_Leak_Rate_and_Leak_Rate. Accessed March 1, 2024.
21. Kumar S, Anton A, D'Ambrosio CM. Sex differences in obstructive sleep apnea. *Clin Chest Med.* 2021;42(3):417-425.
22. McArdle N, King S, Shepherd K, et al. Study of a novel APAP algorithm for the treatment of obstructive sleep apnea in women. *Sleep.* 2015;38(11):1775-1781.
23. Bitter T, Langer C, Vogt J, et al. Sleep-disordered breathing in patients with atrial fibrillation and normal systolic left ventricular function. *Dtsch Arztebl Int.* 2009;106(10):164-170.
24. Thomas RJ, Bianchi MT. Urgent need to improve PAP management: the devil is in two (fixable) details. *J Clin Sleep Med.* 2017;13(5):657-664.

Telemedicine Strategies to Improve PAP Adherence

Michelle T. Cao   ▓   Ashima S. Sahni

Introduction

In 2020 the *Wall Street Journal* published an article titled, "Telemedicine, Once a Hard Sell, Can't Keep Up With Demand," which precisely described how the coronavirus disease 2019 (COVID-19) pandemic has reshaped health care and has brought medicine to the patient's doorstep neatly packaged in the smart phone.[1] In reality, this is a reflection of the changing landscape of medicine from provider-centric to patient-driven care. The American Telemedicine Association elaborates telemedicine as a "means of connecting individuals with their health care providers while fostering safe, convenient, secure and quality care." The American Academy of Sleep Medicine (AASM) recognizes that live interactive telemedicine sessions for sleep disorders are comparable to traditional in-person visits and identifies telemedicine as a means of improving access to care and promoting professionalism by improving care coordination between sleep medicine and other specialities.[2] Telemedicine applications are broadly characterized into four categories.[3,4] This section aims to discuss these four categories and their applications to positive airway pressure (PAP) adherence strategies. The categories are as follows:

1. Synchronous—Real-time visits that could be done by physicians, nurses, or respiratory therapists.
2. Asynchronous visits—The encounter does not happen in real time. This includes electronic messaging, remote monitoring, automated care mechanisms, and self-management platforms.
3. Remote patient monitoring (RPM).
4. Mobile health (mHealth) smart phone application.

Positive Airway Pressure Adherence and Challenges

The definition of *PAP adherence* is arbitrary and predominantly based on the accepted criteria by third-party payer systems. Despite a true acknowledgment of PAP adherence being a moving target and having a clear dose response to clinical outcomes, PAP usage of *less than* 4 hours per night for 70% of nights has been adopted to define PAP non-adherence.[5] Improving PAP adherence has been one of the most challenging aspects of sleep medicine, with adherence ranges varying between 30% and 60% depending on studies reviewed. Because the pattern of PAP usage is established early in the course of treatment, early interventions are critically important in improving outcomes.[6]

To date, not a single factor has stood out that if targeted improves PAP adherence. Thus sleep medicine providers resort to multidimensional approaches[7] to tackle this challenging goal by including behavior and psychological modalities, which have shown sustained improvements in PAP adherence. Psycho-educational interventions include initiating phone follow-ups and providing education on obstructive sleep apnea (OSA) and the benefits of PAP treatment. A limiting factor with education, supportive protocols, and motivational enhancement programs is that they can be labor- and time-intensive for both the patient and the medical provider. In this regard, telemedicine provides an opportunity for efficient and personalized counseling with the same end goal of improving and achieving treatment adherence.

For telemedicine to be accepted by patients, it must be able to deliver safe and effective care and be user-friendly. Parikh and colleagues showed that compared with traditional in-person face-to face-visits, telemedicine via video-conferencing did not significantly alter patient satisfaction scores.[8] A recent study employing telemedicine approaches to OSA management showed that 9 of 10 patients were able to successfully use the online application portal and found it straightforward and innovative. The patients' positive perception of telemedicine included flexibility, time saving, reduced trips to the hospital, and a chance to follow up on therapy closely.[9] This effective and efficient model may also lead to reduction in total health care costs.[10]

Telemedicine Applications for PAP Adherence

Educational, supportive, and behavioral interventions have been shown to improve PAP adherence.[11] Most behavioral interventions are based on principles of decision balancing (one's ability to weigh pros and cons leading to a change)[7] and self-efficacy (one's ability to resort to a change dispute if it is perceived to be difficult).[11,12] Studies have evaluated telemedicine applications on enhanced PAP adherence based on the aforementioned principles. Telemedicine strategies to improve PAP adherence can be divided into synchronous or asynchronous models. Synchronous models incorporate face-to-face interactive virtual visits with sleep medicine providers delivering education and counseling. Synchronous models require scheduling, real-time appointments, and a dedicated time slot. Asynchronous models include remote monitoring and adjustments to therapy, automated motivational phone/text reminders, web-based education, and active interactions with a provider calling the patient by phone or providing patient feedback as a form of encouraging patient engagement (Figure 19.1). Compared with a synchronous model, an asynchronous model is fluid, flexible, and non-stringent.

Telemedicine provides an opportunity to deliver education, provide support, and promote patient engagement on a "virtual" platform. This section aims to discuss "virtual-based" platforms and provide evidence-based data (when available), with acknowledgment that multiple telemedicine-based applications are proprietary and developed by stakeholders of OSA therapy. Virtual platforms also vary in their designs, with many sharing similar aspects on education, data presentation, and patient feedback.

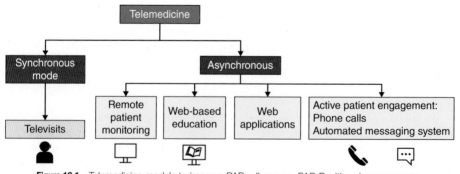

Figure 19.1   Telemedicine models to improve PAP adherence. *PAP,* Positive airway pressure.

WEB-BASED EDUCATION

Prior studies have indicated that patient education is an important variable in improving adherence to PAP therapy. Web-based education programs are an efficient method of delivery in clinical environments with time constraints. Lai and colleagues examined the efficacy of a multicomponent motivational enhancement education program that included web-based education added to usual care to improve continuous positive airway pressure (CPAP) adherence in 100 patients.[13] Usual care was composed of education on the importance of CPAP therapy for OSA. The intervention arm included use of a 25-minute education video, a 20-minute patient-centered interview, and a 10-minute phone follow-up. This model combined a "web-based education" component with "active patient engagement" through questionnaires and phone follow-up. The authors reported positive results with higher daily CPAP usage by 2 hours ($p<0.001$), a fourfold increase in number of patients using CPAP for >70% of days with >4 hours/day ($p<0.001$), and greater improvements in daytime sleepiness.[13]

PATIENT ENGAGEMENT APPLICATIONS

Phone Calls

A systematic review found that the addition of education and motivational programs significantly improves PAP adherence compared with usual care.[14] However, the specific method of delivery, location, and program duration are key factors in the sleep provider's ability to successfully provide this supportive tool to patients. Telemedicine-based programs can bypass the time and location constraints on multiple levels and can be made widely available to a wider audience. Sedkaoui and colleagues conducted a multicenter randomized controlled trial comparing standard support to phone-based coaching sessions (five sessions total) for patients newly initiated on CPAP therapy ($n = 379$).[15] The primary outcome was percentage of patients using CPAP >3 hours/night for 4 months. Compared with standard care, 75% of patients in the phone-based counseling group (coached group) met the primary end point versus 65% in the standard support group. Mean CPAP usage also increased in the coached group by 26 minutes ($p=0.04$).[15] A limiting factor with person-initiated phone-based support is time and staffing resource.

Promotion of patient accountability by collaborative OSA management is an important element in improving PAP adherence. This could be achieved by active patient engagement.[3] One way of doing this is by incorporating a phone interactive voice response system to monitor the patient's self-reported behavior and provide pre-recorded feedback and counseling based on the patient's response. Sparrow and colleagues assessed this method in 250 patients and showed an improvement in CPAP adherence by 1 hour/night at 6 months and 2 hours/night at 12 months when compared with the control arm, though adherence in the control arm was very low.[16] A similar approach by Fox and colleagues showed that care coordinator–driven patient engagement via phone calls based on remotely transmitted CPAP data improved adherence after 3 months (telemedicine arm = 191 minutes/day vs. standard arm = 105 minutes/day; $p=0.006$). This intervention, however, led to an extra hour of care coordinator time, thereby adding additional labor cost.[17] The "HOPES" study aimed to determine whether PAP adherence can be improved by implementing a PAP training strategy during rehabilitation combined with a telemedicine monitoring system in post-stroke patients.[18] In this study, a "PAP" coordinator reviewed the downloaded information from the device every morning and contacted the patient if any of the following data were noted: 90th percentile pressure >16 cm H_2O, mask leakage >24 L/min, use <4 hours, apnea-hypopnea index (AHI) >10 events per hour for three consecutive nights. The authors found that the group with proactive tele-monitored PAP treatment increased hours of usage at the 3-month mark (76 minutes longer per night; $p=0.017$).[18] This positive finding was unfortunately lost at the 1-year mark; however, the study dropout rate was higher at 1 year.

Automated Messaging System

Hwang and colleagues conducted a large randomized clinical trial ($n = 1455$) comparing web-based OSA education (Tel-Ed) versus CPAP tele-monitoring with automated patient feedback (Tel-TM) with a primary end point of 90-day CPAP adherence.[19] Patients were randomized into four arms: usual care, Tel-Ed, Tel-TM, or Tel-Ed plus Tel-TM. Two proprietary programs were utilized for the study (Emmi Solutions, Inc. and U-Sleep, ResMed). The investigators reported that use of CPAP tele-monitoring with automated feedback messaging (Tel-TM) and Tel-TM plus web-based OSA education (Tel-Ed) were superior to usual care ($p=0.0002$). In addition, web-based OSA education (Tel-Ed) alone did not improve PAP adherence. The PAP adherence improvement was observed without extra cost to health care or the patient. Interestingly, post hoc analysis indicated that the U-Sleep effect diminished 3 months after the patient feedback system was "turned off," with a gradual decline in CPAP adherence until it was identical to the non–U-Sleep users. A small subgroup in which the automated messaging was continued showed sustained PAP adherence at the 1-year mark (% days used at 330 to 360 days was 58.4% to 41.1% vs. 48.1% to 43.9%, $p=0.05$). This finding suggests that continuation of messaging in support of PAP usage may be the optimal approach for a sustained long-term response. Additionally, similar to the Lai study,[13] a multicomponent tele-monitoring model proved to be superior to web-based education alone. This important study highlights that accountability (i.e., patient engagement) may be more effective than solo educational interventions in changing behavior and also that increased contact with the sleep provider (even though automated) may be associated with positive feedback and meaningful outcomes. Only a small number of patients refused to receive messages.[19]

WEB APPLICATIONS

Online interactive websites are another virtual platform developed by companies to enhance CPAP adherence (Table 19.1). This platform was studied in a small, randomized study via a

TABLE 19.1 ■ Virtual Platforms and Applications on Targeting PAP Adherence

Virtual Platform	Manufacturer	Designed for Patient or Provider	Data Provided
DreamMapper[21]	Philips Respironics	Patient	Actively engages patients with daily reminders, encouragement messages, troubleshooting advice, and educational content
AirView	ResMed	Provider	A secure, cloud-based system for online monitoring of PAP use and efficacy
MyAir[22]	ResMed	Patient	This user-friendly web program allows patients to track their nightly sleep data and provides interactive coaching
U-Sleep[23]	ResMed	Patient and provider	Provides active feedback by processing PAP data (automatically and remotely collected) Sends automated messages encouraging use Assists in identifying issues with PAP usage
PAMS (Patient Adherence Management Service)[24]	Philips Respironics	Patient and provider	Provides a "personal" coach to help educate, motivate, and manage PAP therapy, with escalation to respiratory therapy when clinically appropriate Provides centralized care with remote tele-monitoring that might help in the private sector

PAP, Positive airway pressure.

website (MyCPAP) that consisted of a virtual learning center, access to patient-friendly usage reports, patient tracking forms including sleepiness scales, interactive PAP usage manual videos, and education forms on common CPAP issues and solutions.[20] This model showed increased CPAP adherence when compared with usual care by 1 hour at 2 months with sustained effect at 4 months.

Manufacturers of PAP devices have developed online programs aimed at patient engagement toward the patient's own "sleep health." These programs capture overnight data on PAP usage and provide daily feedback in the form of positive reinforcement and/or supportive reminders to the user (patient). *MyAir* is an online support program and smart phone app developed by ResMed that automatically sends data from the patient's PAP device to a computer or mobile phone in the form of a sleep score (the higher the score, the more effective hours on PAP therapy). In a retrospective review, the *MyAir* program showed improved PAP adherence when compared with usual care and was most significant in patients who "struggled" with CPAP adherence.[22] The *MyAir* app is password protected and provides information to the patient in terms of hours of usage, AHI, and mask leak. Patients get real-time feedback, appreciation messages, reinforcement messages, and personalized coaching.

The web-based *U-Sleep*, developed by ResMed, is an online program that takes a step further by connecting the patient's PAP usage information with the sleep provider. *U-Sleep* monitors PAP adherence and notifies the medical provider if a patient seems to be struggling with usage and is at risk of not meeting 90-day adherence. *U-Sleep* led to a reduced provider coaching labor requirement (58.3 ± 25 vs. 23.9 ± 26 minutes, 59% reduction; $p<0.0001$), though the CPAP adherence was no different than that of the control arm, partially due to increase in CPAP adherence equally in both arms.[23]

Another proprietary program called *PAMS* (*Patient Adherence Management Service*; Philips Respironics) is a cloud-based sleep coach (CBSC)[24] model based on protocol-driven live phone contact with the patient when initiating PAP therapy (for 30 days). PAMS improved initial 90-day adherence when compared with standard care (SC: respiratory therapist led CPAP setup + remote tele-monitoring + elective use of mobile adherence feedback application) in a group of 250 patients at a Veterans Affairs Health Care. At 90 days, the percentage of days with ≥4 hours of PAP use was higher in the PAMS group (SC: 48.1 ± 36.8% vs. SC + CBSC: 57.9 ± 3 5.4%, $p=0.032$). In the PAMS program, "sleep coaches" made contact with the patient in the early phases of CPAP initiation to monitor adherence, provided motivational enhancement, and escalated issues related to CPAP to the sleep provider or respiratory therapist. Patients also utilized *DreamMapper*, a mobile app (Philips Respironics), that provided positive feedback based on PAP usage data.

REMOTE MONITORING

Other benefits of telemedicine monitoring include reduction in delay to first intervention[25] and reduction in the rate of therapy termination.[26] Telemedicine allows remote monitoring of PAP devices and allows the provider to determine if a device is effectively treating the underlying sleep apnea condition. For example, through remote monitoring, various types of residual apneas can be detected. Analysis of a large tele-monitored database showed emergence of clinical phenotypes of central sleep apnea (CSA) during the course of CPAP therapy, highlighting higher risk of therapy termination due to treatment-emergent CSA ($p<0.001$). Thus tele-monitoring provides an opportunity for early intervention by timely detection of central apneas, thereby preventing premature termination of CPAP therapy and possibly enhancing long-term CPAP adherence.[27] Anttalainen and colleagues compared remote PAP monitoring versus usual care during the habituation phase of CPAP initiation for OSA. The authors reported that compared with usual care, remote monitoring was able to save nursing time and resources (median 39 vs. 58 minutes per patient, $p<0.001$), highlighting the potential positive impact of remote monitoring on limited health care resources and time.[28]

CPAP BUDDY SYSTEM

There are online communities hosted by medical societies or device manufacturers. Examples include "myapnea.org" developed by the AASM and "waketosleep.com" developed by ResMed Inc. Though these portals have not been studied in clinical trials, an interesting small pilot study showed increased user satisfaction and higher CPAP adherence through use of a human buddy system.[29] In this prospective randomized study, the peer buddy system group (patient partnering with an experienced CPAP user, "peer buddy") had significantly higher satisfaction scores and CPAP adherence compared with usual care at the 3-month mark. Larger studies would be valuable to determine important outcomes including long-term effectiveness and cost-effectiveness.

Integration of Electronic Health Records With Remote Tele-monitoring Platforms

Despite the explosion of technological advancement in cloud-based platforms and remote monitoring of PAP therapy, a limitation is lack or ease of integration between the virtual-based platforms and the electronic medical records (EMRs).[30] Web-based programs are proprietary and therefore come with legal and logistical challenges. However, in a perfect world, the integration of remote monitoring and virtual data acquisition into EMR can potentially identify high-risk non-adherent patient populations and provide support to improve outcomes in an efficient and effective way. High-risk groups can be identified based on factors including ethnicity, social economic status, education level, personality types,[31] subjective characteristics such as daytime sleepiness questionnaires, and the presence or absence of claustrophobia. Hwang and colleagues proposed a comprehensive end-to-end care integration of electronic health records with PAP device data, polysomnograms results, and tele-monitoring platforms that incorporate patient-provider interchange via web-based education/questionnaires.[3] Tan and colleagues showed a successful model of integration of EMR and remote tele-monitoring that alerted patients and sleep providers on PAP adherence statistics.[32]

Summary

Telemedicine platforms can be successfully applied to PAP adherence strategies through a combination of web-based education, web applications, automatic messaging systems providing positive feedback to the patient, and promoting patient engagement in improving the patient's own sleep health. Telemedicine models for PAP adherence may prove to be less labor intensive, improves efficiency, and is cost-effective. A meta-analysis ($n = 5429$ adults with OSA) investigated the effectiveness of a broad range of "eHealth" interventions in improving CPAP treatment adherence and showed significant improvements in adherence rate in the initial months of therapy initiation when compared with usual care. Subgroup analysis did not review differences in regard to type of eHealth intervention or a single versus combination of interventions.[33]

Uncertainty exists in regard to specific interventions, including timing/duration/intensity of the intervention along with cost-effectiveness. Long-term PAP adherence is questionable as most studies evaluated adherence up to 3 months. Gender, age, and socioeconomic/demographic issues have not been addressed in the trials, which may hamper the widespread application of telemedicine. Cost-effectiveness is debatable, though one can argue that the added cost of this intervention can be offset by improved CPAP adherence reducing health care cost by avoiding cardiovascular events if this trend translates into long-term CPAP adherence.[34] Also, practical implications must be considered regarding local payment of teleservices along with the investment needed for successful implication of this in terms of infrastructure and manpower. Future studies should target direct comparisons of different telemedicine strategies and long-term effectiveness of virtual-based interventions in improving PAP treatment adherence. PAP adherence strategies through virtual platforms are here to stay, and opportunities exist for growth and improvement.

References

1. Topol EJ. The future of medicine is in your smartphone. *Wall Street Journal*. 2015. Available at: http://www.wsj.com/articles/the-future-of-medicine-is-in-yoursmartphone-1420828632. Accessed March 1, 2024. (Telemedicine, Once a Hard Sell, Can't Keep Up With Demand - WSJ).
2. Singh J, Badr MS, Diebert W, et al. American Academy of Sleep Medicine (AASM) position paper for the use of telemedicine for the diagnosis and treatment of sleep disorders. *J Clin Sleep Med*. 2015;11(10):1187-1198.
3. Hwang D. Monitoring progress and adherence with positive airway pressure therapy for obstructive sleep apnea: the roles of telemedicine and mobile health applications. *Sleep Med Clin*. 2016;11:161-171.
4. Singh J, Keer N. Overview of telemedicine and sleep disorders. *Sleep Med Clin*. 2020;15(3):341-346.
5. Sunwood BY, Light M, Malhotra A. Strategies to augment adherence in the management of sleep-disordered breathing. *Respirology*. 2020;25:363-371.
6. Weaver TE, Sawyer AM. Adherence to continuous positive airway pressure treatment for obstructive sleep apnoea: implications for future interventions. *Indian J Med Res*. 2010;131:245-258.
7. Sawyer AM, Gooneratne NS, Marcus CL, et al. A systematic review of CPAP adherence across age groups: clinical and empiric insights for developing CPAP adherence interventions. *Sleep Med Rev*. 2011;15:343-356.
8. Parikh R, Touvelle MN, Wang H, et al. Sleep telemedicine: patient satisfaction and treatment adherence. *Telemed J E Health*. 2011;17:609-614.
9. Garmendia O, Suarez-Giron MC, Torres M, Montserrat JM. Telemedicine in sleep apnea: a simple approach for nasal pressure treatment. *Arch Bronconeumol (Engl Ed)*. 2018;54(9):491-492.
10. Isetta V, Negrin MA, Monasterio C, et al. A Bayesian cost-effectiveness analysis of a telemedicine-based strategy for the management of sleep apnea: a multicentre randomised controlled trial. *Thorax*. 2015;70:1054-1061.
11. Wozniak DR, Lasserson TJ, Smith I. Educational, supportive and behavioural interventions to improve usage of continuous positive airway pressure machines in adults with obstructive sleep apnoea. *Cochrane Database Syst Rev*. 2014;(1):CD007736.
12. Sawyer AM, Deatrick JA, Kuna ST, et al. Differences in perceptions of the diagnosis and treatment of obstructive sleep apnea and continuous positive airway pressure therapy among adherer and nonadherence. *Qual Health Res*. 2010;20:873-892.
13. Lai AYK, Fong DYT, Lam JCM, et al. The efficacy of a brief motivational enhancement education program on CPAP adherence in OSA: a randomized controlled trial. *Chest*. 2014;146:600-610.
14. Smith I, Nadig V, Lasserson TJ. Educational, supportive, and behavioral interventions to improve usage of continuous positive airway pressure machines for adults with obstructive sleep apnea. *Cochrane Database Syst Rev*. 2009;(2):CD007736.
15. Sedkaoui K, Leseux L, Pontier S, et al. Efficiency of a phone coaching program on adherence to continuous positive airway pressure in sleep apnea hypopnea syndrome: a randomized trial. *BMC Pulm Med*. 2015;15:102.
16. Sparrow D, Aloia M, Demolles DA, et al. A telemedicine intervention to improve adherence to continuous positive airway pressure: a randomized controlled trial. *Thorax*. 2010;65:1061-1066.
17. Fox N, Hirsch-Allen AJ, Goodfellow E, et al. The impact of a telemedicine monitoring system on positive airway pressure adherence in patients with obstructive sleep apnea: a randomized controlled trial. *Sleep*. 2012;35:477-481.
18. Kotzian ST, Saletu MT, Schwarzinger A, et al. Proactive telemedicine monitoring of sleep apnea treatment improves adherence in people with stroke—a randomized controlled trial (HOPES study). *Sleep Med*. 2019;64:48-55.
19. Hwang D, Chang JW, Benjafield AV, et al. Effect of telemedicine education and telemonitoring on continuous positive airway pressure adherence. The Tele-OSA randomized trial. *Am J Respir Crit Care Med*. 2018;197(1):117-126.

20. Stepnowsky C, Edwards C, Zamora T, et al. Patient perspective on use of an interactive website for sleep apnea. *Int J Telemed Appl.* 2013;2013:239382.
21. Hardy W, Powers J, Jasko JG, et al. *SleepMapper. A Mobile Application and Website to Engage Sleep Apnea Patients in PAP Therapy and Improve Adherence to Treatment.* https://www.philips.us/sleepmapper. Accessed March 1, 2024.
22. Malhotra A, Crocker ME, Willes L, et al. Patient engagement using new technology to improve adherence to positive airway pressure therapy. *Chest.* 2018;153(4):843-850.
23. Munafo D, Hevener W, Crocker M, et al. A telehealth program for CPAP adherence reduces labor and yields similar adherence and efficacy when compared to standard of care. *Sleep Breath.* 2016;20:777-785.
24. Berry RB, Beck E, Jasko JG. Effect of cloud-based sleep coaches on positive airway pressure adherence. *J Clin Sleep Med.* 2020;16(4):553-562.
25. Hoet F, Libert W, Sanida C, et al. Telemonitoring in continuous positive airway pressure-treated patients improves delay to first intervention and early compliance: a randomized trial. *Sleep Med.* 2017;39:77-83.
26. Woehrle H, Ficker JH, Graml A, et al. Telemedicine-based proactive patient management during positive airway pressure therapy: impact on therapy termination rate. *Somnologie (Berl).* 2017;21(2):121-127.
27. Liu D, Armitstead J, Benjafield A, et al. Trajectories of emergent central sleep apnea during CPAP therapy. *Chest.* 2017;152(4):751–760. S0012-3692:31079-6.
28. Anttalainen U, Melkko S, Hakko S, et al. Telemonitoring of CPAP therapy may save nursing time. *Sleep Breath.* 2016;20:1209-1215.
29. Parthasarathy S, Wendel C, Haynes PL, et al. A pilot study of CPAP adherence promotion by peer buddies with sleep apnea. *J Clin Sleep Med.* 2013;9(6):543-550.
30. Bottaz-Bosson G, Midelet A, Mendelson M, et al. Remote monitoring of positive airway pressure data: challenges, pitfalls, and strategies to consider for optimal data science applications. *Chest.* 2023;163(5):1279-1291.
31. Dieltjens M, Vanderveken OM, Van den Bosch D, et al. Impact of type D personality on adherence to oral appliance therapy for sleep-disordered breathing. *Sleep Breath.* 2013;17:985-991.
32. Tan M, Keenan B, Staley B, et al. Using an Electronic Health Record (EHR) to identify chronic CPAP users with abnormal HL7 CPAP data. *Sleep.* 2018;41(1):402.
33. Aardoom JJ, Loheide-Niesmann L, Ossebaard HC, et al. Effectiveness of eHealth interventions in improving treatment adherence for adults with obstructive sleep apnea: meta-analytic review. *J Med Internet Res.* 2020;22(2):e16972.
34. Bouloukaki I, Giannadaki K, Mermigkis C, et al. Intensive versus standard follow-up to improve continuous positive airway pressure compliance. *Eur Respir J.* 2014;44:1262-1274.

CHAPTER 20

Mask Fitting and Machine Setups

Michelle T. Cao ■ Ashima S. Sahni

Introduction

The term *telemedicine* was coined in 1970 with the definition of providing "healing at a distance."[1] Telemedicine has since evolved to a broad inclusive definition. The World Health Organization (WHO) defines *telehealth* as "delivery of health care services, where patients and providers are separated by distance." Telehealth can contribute to achieving universal health coverage by improving patient access to quality and cost-effective health care services wherever they may be. It is particularly valuable for patients who reside in remote areas, including vulnerable groups and the aging population.[2] With the projected physician shortage, telemedicine can provide efficient, cost-effective, and accessible alternatives to traditional in-person clinical care, while ensuring patient privacy. This remote care model proved to be a "silver lining" during the coronavirus disease 2019 (COVID-19) pandemic and exponentially grew in ways that the medical field has never seen before.

Based on the American Academy of Sleep Medicine (AASM) 2015 position statement "Use of Telemedicine for the Diagnosis and Treatment of Sleep Disorders,"[3] continuous positive airway pressure (CPAP) device setup by video and online education can be considered an acceptable alternative to face-to-face interaction, making this an attractive alternative for remote CPAP device setups and mask fittings. These venues can be achieved by various tele-video conferences, individually or in group settings.[4]

Since the invention of CPAP in 1981, nasal mask interface was the initial mode of delivery of positive airway pressure (PAP) therapy. Over time, manufacturers have developed various PAP interfaces including oronasal (full-face) masks, nasal masks, nasal pillows, and total face masks. Recognizing the importance of mask fit to achieving PAP adherence and efficacy, the American Thoracic Society (ATS) published a workshop report highlighting the importance of mask selection for CPAP therapy as an important obstructive sleep apnea (OSA)-related outcome.[5]

Since the onset of the COVID-19 pandemic, manufacturers of PAP equipment have quickly pivoted to overcome obstacles created by social distancing and implemented innovative ideas on safe PAP device setups and mask fittings, although these practices are based on practical applications rather than sound scientific evidence. Some novel interventions include mask-fitting facial recognition software, use of mask sizers via video calls, and mask fit packs containing several cushion sizes. This section aims to review virtual-based programs for PAP device setup and mask fitting, recognizing that the programs are proprietary to stakeholders including PAP device manufacturers, while there is little evidence on treatment effectiveness or improved PAP adherence.

Positive Airway Pressure Device Setup

In the United States, PAP device setups are primarily the responsibility of durable medical equipment (DME) providers and performed in-person, either individually or in group settings. However, the COVID-19 pandemic posed challenges and encouraged sleep medicine stakeholders to develop novel ideas for device setups in a practical and safe environment.[6] Like the rest of medicine, DME providers turned to online platforms (e.g., Zoom, FaceTime, Skype, Webex) to continue to deliver

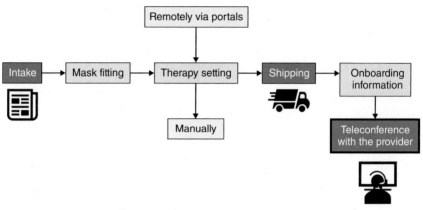

Figure 20.1   Checklist for PAP device setup.

care and in an efficient manner. In the "virtual" workflow, the PAP device is pre-programmed based on the provider's prescription, shipped to the patient's home, and then instructions for setup are provided via real-time video-conferencing between DME staff and the patient. Manufacturers of PAP equipment have also come up with checklists (Figure 20.1) for DME providers to ensure satisfactory device setups.

POSITIVE AIRWAY PRESSURE MASK FITTING

Proper mask fitting is critical in the first weeks of CPAP therapy as long-term adherence is determined during this time. Telemedicine provides a unique and timely opportunity for the patient and provider in which mask fitting and education can be implemented in an efficient and cost-effective way. This approach can also encourage proactive self-management, promote a patient-centered approach, and increase partner participation in mask selection.[7]

The COVID-19 pandemic has led to rapid adoption of virtual PAP mask-fitting programs through video-conferencing. Manufacturers of PAP equipment developed fit packs and mask-fitting software for remote implementation of mask fitting. These programs are new to the field and have not been studied or compared with traditional mask-fitting programs (in-person, hands-on approach). Data on cost-effectiveness and PAP adherence are not available with these "remote" programs. Remote mask-fitting programs offer a safe environment while providing multiple options for patients. For example, ResMed's (San Diego, California) remote device and mask setup kit includes a pre-programmed CPAP device and mask interface based on the selection and measurements, multiple mask size cushions, patient education sheet, and equipment company contact information.[8]

Virtual Platforms

The following are examples of remote mask-fitting programs that have been developed by stakeholders of PAP therapy. We aim to review the programs without a preference for one over another. As evidence-based approaches or practices are not available, we elected to describe several widely used telemedicine-based options.

FIT PACKS

Fit packs, as the name indicates, contain multiple cushion sizes of the same mask style to reduce the need for sterilization and re-delivery. Fit packs aid in the implementation of telehealth technology for PAP mask fitting in a safe manner by providing patients with options right at their fingertips during video-conferencing.

- ■ "DreamWear" fit packs (Philips Respironics): provides headgear, frame, and multi-sized cushions (extra-small, small, medium, large, wide) to reduce re-delivery cost and expedite time to initiation of the PAP therapy. Each pack comes with fitting instructions and sizing gauge for proper fit. Patients can size and refit on their own in the convenience of their home. This method can promote patient engagement of PAP therapy.
- ■ "Starter pack" (ResMed) comes in multi-sized mask cushions with fitting instructions and a sizing gauge to help with proper fit. The manufacturing company also developed posters categorizing the masks based on various body positions during sleep, materials used, and footprint on the face to help with better mask selection.

REMOTE FACIAL SCANNING

The new three-dimensional (3D) mask selector (Philips Respironics) provides patients with a self-scanning solution to find the correct fitting mask via the patient's own digital device. This is a novel technique that can potentially eliminate the need for in-person, hands-on mask-fitting sessions. It is also the first program to provide a "custom fit" mask and is a step toward personalized telemedicine (https://www.youtube.com/watch?time_continue=8&v=99b3np0G_ps&feature=emb_log).

ResMed developed a similar program called *MaskSelector* that creates a unique link that is sent to patients via text or email. This functions as a personal web-based patient portal by allowing patients to select the optimal mask and size. The program aims to provide a personalized process based on answers to several key questions including the ability of the patient to put headgear over the head, history of skin irritation, nasal dryness, use of eyeglass, intimacy, and insomnia tendencies. This is followed by a measuring tool to determine nose width, face height, and nose depth. Subsequently, the mask selection is sent to the patient. This program can also be used by patients who do not have access to a web camera. It allows for automated workflow, which can improve efficiency.

If the patient or clinician cannot access or does not want to use a mask selector, the program can also provide the patient with a sizing template and instructions (https://ap.resmed.com/en/knowledge/how-do-i-know-what-size-cpap-mask-i-need). In addition, ResMed has developed a web-based portfolio approach to mask selection to simplify the process for both clinicians and patients (https://document.resmed.com/en-us/documents/products/sleep/resmed-guidebook_remote-cpap-setups_mask-selection_amer_eng.pdf).

Fit packs and remote mask fitting are advantageous in providing "remote" setups; however, providers should be cognizant of factors that may play a role in proper-fitting mask selection. Proper mask fitting and patient comfort are often determined by a combination of physical and psychological challenges. Similar to in-person mask-fitting sessions, these factors will need to be addressed in virtual platforms.[9]

1. Patient specific factors: facial morphology, age, sleep habits/position, gender
2. Breathing patterns: nose versus mouth breathing and nasal symptoms
3. Frequency and length of PAP usage
4. Claustrophobia: home-based mask desensitization may need to be implemented
5. Trial of the mask with the prescribed PAP therapy to ensure proper mask fit and help in verification and addressing mask leak

PATIENT-SPECIFIC FACTORS

The patient's facial morphology plays an important role in mask fitting. A randomized controlled study looking at demographic data, Nasal Obstruction Symptom Evaluation (NOSE) scores, and craniofacial measurements in an Asian cohort concluded that patients with superior adherence to an oronasal mask had less nasal obstruction (based on the NOSE score) and a proportionally increased chin lower-lip distance to mid-face width, highlighting the importance of facial measurements in finding an appropriate mask.[10] With virtual mask fitting, facial measurements can be carried out by the patient with guidance from a sleep technician. Facial measurement instructions (video or print) can be provided to patients prior to the video session.

Facial 3D scanning is another promising option that can "photograph" a patient's specific facial configuration including bony prominences, angle of nose, and tissue thickness, features that can be overlooked by sizing template due to its two-dimensional (2D) nature.[9] Evidence is lacking to support this option, but 3D facial scanning theoretically would be able to offer personalized "custom-made" mask options. Remote mask-fitting online tools may be a step closer to personalized 3D scanning. 3D photography and use of patient-specific computer-aided designs like 3D CAD software (e.g., Mimics, Materialise, Belgium) have precedence in pediatric patients with craniofacial abnormalities with improvement in mask comfort, leaks, and residual apnea indexes, though this technology is limited by lack of clinical trials showing improved efficacy over traditional in-person mask fit.[11-13]

BREATHING PATTERNS

The debate on the effectiveness of oronasal versus nasal masks is worth mentioning. Despite the clear benefit of a nasal mask over an oronasal mask and evidence that self-reported breathing patterns do not translate to objective metrics, a patient endorsing mouth breathing during a mask-fitting session will likely be offered an oronasal mask.[14] Prior evidence shows that patients endorsing mouth breathing usually will switch to nasal breathing when placed on a nasal mask.[15] Moreover, oronasal masks are associated with increased upper airway obstruction due to neutralization of the splinting effect of the upper airway (i.e., pushing the soft palate against the tongue) and posterior displacement of the mandible.[16,17] Interestingly, when the mouth was taped shut, the airway narrowing with an oronasal mask was not seen, which may allude to the various forms of OSA endotypes affecting the site(s) of upper airway obstruction.[16,18] Another issue with oronasal masks is higher PAP pressure requirements due to the iatrogenic pharyngeal narrowing. This may be associated with reduced PAP adherence as seen in the meta-analysis.[19,20]

Patient satisfaction is higher with the use of nasal masks.[21] In a randomized crossover study conducted in an Asian cohort with moderate to severe sleep apnea, use of a nasal mask was associated with better adherence when compared with use of an oronasal mask (3.96 ± 2.26 hours/night vs. 3.26 ± 2.18 hours/night; $p<0.001$) and nasal pillows (3.96 ± 2.26 hours/night vs. 3.48 ± 2.20 hours/night; $p=0.007$). Higher residual apnea-hypopnea index (AHI) was noted with an oronasal mask when compared with a nasal mask and nasal pillow.[10] A retrospective analysis by Schell and colleagues showed the highest adherence in subgroups on nasal pillows followed by nasal masks when compared with mouth-covering interfaces (oronasal) despite the presence of rhino-sinusal symptoms. Thus it is debatable whether the presence of rhinosinusitis would predict more favorable outcomes with the use of an oronasal mask.[22]

There are limited data between nasal pillows and nasal interfaces. A small study comparing nasal pillows to standard nasal masks showed no significant differences in PAP adherence and AHI after 4 weeks of therapy. Most patients found nasal pillows to be more comfortable with less pressure on the face, although this did not reach statistical significance.[23] The debate clearly emphasizes the need for more personalized mask selection and debunking the approach of "one mask fits all" or "oronasal mask" as the default choice in the presence of mouth breathing.

ADDRESSING MASK LEAK

Mask leaks may limit patient comfort and consequently hamper PAP adherence. Multiple factors can contribute to a high leak, including poor mask seal or mouth breathing. Nasal masks provide PAP when there is coupling of the tongue with the soft palate. Once this coupling is lost, due to

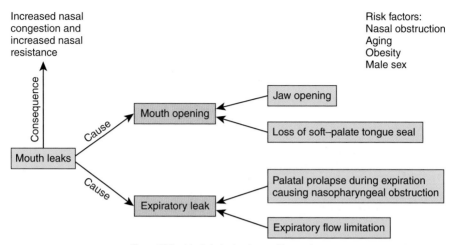

Figure 20.2 Mask leak due to mouth opening.

prolapse of the soft palate or mouth opening, leaks are inevitable.[24] Thus mouth leaks could be due to mouth opening or expiratory leaks (Figure 20.2). Interventions for mouth leak include addition of a chin strap, treatment of nasal obstruction, and/or addition of heated humidification. Analysis of PAP download with graphical representation of air leaks can provide vital information in order to differentiate between mouth leak versus mask leak. A sawtooth pattern would suggest mouth leak.[25] Therefore, it is important, even after selecting a mask based on the online software with telemedicine approach, that the sleep technician or respiratory therapist requests that the patient wear the mask with the PAP to measure the leak and identify the source of the leak based on the patient's feedback or based on the leak pattern from the PAP download.

Summary

Sleep medicine providers must be aware of the technical advantages as well as limitations related to PAP device setups and mask fitting in a virtual platform. Demographic factors including age, gender, and body mass index; anatomical profile including nasal obstruction, pharyngeal sensitivity and shape, dentition, central fat distribution, body position, and sleep stage; and PAP pressure contribute to a successful PAP setup and mask fit. These factors must be taken into account via a virtual platform.[26]

Future Directions

Telemedicine strategies such as fit packs and remote online tools for mask fitting have helped sleep medicine providers care for patients suffering from sleep apnea during the health care crisis posed by the COVID-19 pandemic. The virtual platform has grown exponentially, and it is unlikely to halt. Proper setup of PAP devices and mask fittings via a virtual platform can improve access, treatment efficiency, adherence, and patient-treating provider satisfaction. An important hurdle for widespread implementation of remote PAP setups is depersonalization and dehumanization of the process, which is considered vital in avoiding errors. Therefore, ease of communication between the provider and patient along with ensuring that protocols and checkpoints in the delivery system via telemedicine are well set up are vital and much needed for the long-term viability of this platform. 3D face scanning and 3D custom mask printing are promising approaches and a step closer to personalized sleep medicine via the virtual platform. The field is wide open for future telemedicine-based programs and pathways in this largely uncharted territory.

References

1. Strehle EM, Shabde N. One hundred years of telemedicine: does this new technology have a place in pediatrics? *Arch Dis Child.* 2006;91(12):956-959.
2. Health World Organization *A Health Telematics Policy in Support of WHO's Health-for-All Strategy for Global Health Development: A Report of the WHO Group Consultation on Health Telematics, 11-16 December, Geneva, 1997.* http://www.who.int/iris/handle/10665/63857, 1998. Accessed March 1, 2024.
3. Singh J, Badr MS, Diebert W, et al. American Academy of Sleep Medicine (AASM) position paper for the use of telemedicine for the diagnosis and treatment of sleep disorders. *J Clin Sleep Med.* 2015;11(10): 1187-1198.
4. Schutte-Rodin S. Telehealth, telemedicine, and obstructive sleep apnea. *Sleep Med Clin.* 2020;15(3):359-375.
5. Genta PR, Kaminska M, Edwards BA, et al. The importance of mask selection on continuous positive airway pressure outcomes for obstructive sleep apnea. An Official American Thoracic Society Workshop Report. *Ann Am Thorac Soc.* 2020;17(10):1177-1185.
6. Orbea CP, Dupuy-McCaulry KL, Morgentahler T. Prevalence and sources of errors in positive airway pressure therapy provisioning. *J Clin Sleep Med.* 2019;15(5):697-704.
7. Free C, Phillips G, Galli L, et al. The effectiveness of mobile-health technology-based health behaviour change or disease management interventions for health care consumers: a systematic review. *PLoS Med.* 2013;10(1):e1001362.
8. *Home Delivery & Remote Setup Checklist.* Available at: https://document.resmed.com/en-us/documents/products/sleep/resmed_remote-setup-checklist_amer_eng.pdf. Accessed March 1, 2024.
9. Ma Z, Drinnan M, Hyde P, Munguia J. Mask interface for continuous positive airway pressure therapy: selection and design considerations. *Expert Rev Med Devices.* 2018;15(10):725-733.
10. Goh KJ, Soh RY, Leow LC, et al. Choosing the right mask for your Asian patient with sleep apnoea: a randomized, crossover trial of CPAP interfaces. *Respirology.* 2019;24(3):278-285.
11. Morrison R, Van Koevering K, Nasser H, et al. Personalized 3D-printed CPAP masks improve CPAP effectiveness in children with OSA and craniofacial anomalies. Proceedings of the Combined Otolaryngology Spring Meetings; Boston, MA, USA. April 22-26, 2015.
12. Willox M, Metherall P, Jeays-Ward K, et al. Custom-made 3D printed masks for children using non-invasive ventilation: a feasibility study of production method and testing of outcomes in adult volunteers. *J Med Eng Technol.* 2020;44(5):213-223.
13. Custom RS. *3-D Printed Noninvasive Ventilation Mask for Children.* Cincinnati, US: Children's Hospital Medical Center; 2016. Available at: https://clinicaltrials.gov/ct2/show/NCT02896751. Accessed March 1, 2024.
14. Nascimento JA, Genta PR, Fernandes PHS, et al. Predictors of oronasal breathing among obstructive sleep apnea patients and controls. *J Appl Physiol (1985).* 2019;127(6):1579-1585.
15. Bachour A, Maasilta P. Mouth breathing compromises adherence to nasal continuous positive airway pressure therapy. *Chest.* 2004;126(40):1248-1254.
16. Kaminska M, Montpetit A, Mathieu A, et al. Higher effective oronasal versus nasal continuous positive airway pressure in obstructive sleep apnea: effect of mandibular stabilization. *Can Respir J.* 2014;21(4): 234-238.
17. Ng JR, Aiyappan V, Mercer J, et al. Choosing an oronasal mask to deliver continuous positive airway pressure may cause more upper airway obstruction or lead to higher continuous positive airway pressure requirements than a nasal mask in some patients: a case series. *J Clin Sleep Med.* 2016;12(9):1227-1232.
18. Madeiro F, Andrade RGS, Piccin VS, et al. Transmission of oral pressure compromises oronasal CPAP efficacy in the treatment of OSA. *Chest.* 2019;156(6):1187-1194.
19. Patil SP, Ayappa IA, Caples SM, et al. Treatment of adult obstructive sleep apnea with positive airway pressure: an American Academy of Sleep Medicine systematic review, meta-analysis, and GRADE assessment. *J Clin Sleep Med.* 2019;15(2):301-334.
20. Andrade RGS, Viana FM, Nascimento JA, et al. Nasal vs oronasal CPAP for OSA treatment: a meta-analysis. *Chest.* 2018;153(3):665-674.
21. Mortimore IL, Whittle AT, Douglas NJ. Comparison of nose and face mask CPAP therapy for sleep apnoea. *Thorax.* 1998;53(4):290-292.
22. Schell AE, Soose RJ. Positive airway pressure adherence and mask interface in the setting of sinonasal symptoms. *Laryngoscope.* 2017;127(10):2418-2422.

23. Ryan S, Garvey JF, Swan V, et al. Nasal pillows as an alternative interface in patients with obstructive sleep apnoea syndrome initiating continuous positive airway pressure therapy. *J Sleep Res.* 2011;20(2): 367-373.
24. Azarbarzin A, Sands SA, Marques M, et al. Palatal prolapse as a signature of expiratory flow limitation and inspiratory palatal collapse in patients with obstructive sleep apnoea. *Eur Respir J.* 2018;51(2):1701419.
25. Bachour A, Avellan-Hietanen H, Palotie T, Virkkula P. Practical aspects of interface application in CPAP treatment. *Can Respir J.* 2019;2019:7215258.
26. Lebret M, Martinot JB, Arnol N, et al. Factors contributing to unintentional leak during CPAP treatment: a systematic review. *Chest.* 2017;151(3):707-719.

CHAPTER 21

Consumer Sleep Technology

Seema Khosla ■ Sharon Schutte-Rodin

Background

As sleep telemedicine experienced rapid growth during the coronavirus disease 2019 (COVID-19) pandemic, so too did consumer sleep technology (CST). Health became a priority with a focus on how best to avoid illness. Along with proper exercise and nutrition, a newly founded appreciation for the importance of sleep health drove consumers to try to quantify and improve their own sleep. The Pew Research Center found that one in five Americans making more than $75,000/year wore a fitness tracker.[1] This was based on data collected in 2019. Since that time, wearable technology shipments increased by 24% in 2020.[2]

CST has increased its presence in our sleep clinics as well. Clinicians must determine (1) if they will incorporate the data from CST into their decision-making process, (2) if they will review these data during the clinic visit or asynchronously between visits, (3) how to manage the time spent analyzing these data, (4) how to assess the validity of these data, (5) if they will use these data in the process of clinical decision making, and (6) how to communicate this information to their patients. Although CST should not be used in direct clinical decision making, CST may raise clinical suspicions. For example, CST data documenting frequent snoring or a high apnea-hypopnea index (AHI) may influence a clinician's suspicion to pursue apnea testing but not to directly order continuous positive airway pressure (CPAP).

What Is Consumer Sleep Technology?

In 2018, the American Academy of Sleep Medicine (AASM) released a position statement and defined CST as non-prescription devices directly marketed to consumers that may make an assertion to perform sleep monitoring, tracking, or sleep-related interventions.[3] There are three major categories of CST: *application* (app; a program that interfaces with a mobile device and is often paired with other devices), *wearable* (device worn on the body that tracks movement and other physiology), and *nearable* (device placed near but not on the body that also tracks movement and other physiology). These devices often use an accelerometer (either on the device or on the mobile device) and can incorporate sound or sound waves (from the microphone or other wearable or nearable sensors) and/or movement to provide an estimate of sleep, wakefulness, and activity. Some are rudimentary, while others are more complex and purport to stage sleep with clinical accuracy. Their purposes often overlap between tracking sleep and providing guidance/therapy to improve sleep. More recently, some CST devices have added additional sensors such as pulse oximetry, photoplethysmography (PPG), and temperature tracking, and some have incorporated artificial intelligence and machine learning (AI/ML) to provide added physiological and sleep data outputs. Although rapid CST technology innovations may have outpaced scientific evidence, some claimed uses have now advanced from informational to actionable and even therapeutic for some devices/apps and are awaiting review by the U.S. Food and Drug Administration (FDA) for clinical uses.

Clinicians are left to determine whether or not there is a role for CST in clinical practice. Dr. Matt Bianchi coined the term *off-PAP sleep time*.[4] This term refers to sleep that occurs in patients who currently use PAP therapy and who experience sleep episodes outside of their normal PAP usage time. This information has not previously been captured through PAP therapy (unless patients use PAP when they take a nap) and can provide objective data suggesting that patients may be sleepier than initially reported. Reviewing CST data in the course of a clinic visit may reveal episodes of sleep not previously captured using PAP download data. Patients may be attempting to treat residual hypersomnolence by napping without recognizing that perhaps another underlying sleep disorder may exist. This information may also supplement conversations in clinic around proper sleep hygiene, sleep timing, and sleep duration.

How Should We Use Consumer Sleep Technology?

Beyond using CST to determine sleep times, CST may be helpful to determine residual snoring or circadian rhythm disorders. Unlike actigraphy tracking of 2-week sleep, CST may allow for longitudinal assessment of sleep timing and duration. A recent study published in *Sleep* demonstrated that the accuracy of certain wearable devices may be superior to actigraphy on sleep/wake performance measures.[5] This has profound implications on the use of CST in a clinical practice. For CST that utilizes advanced AI/ML algorithms and added sensors such as pulse oximetry, PPG, or temperature tracking, some CST may claim to add sleep outputs such as AHI and/or sleep staging reports. It is important to note that often these outputs have not been validated and are not equivalent to the data represented by the same terms in the context of a polysomnography (PSG) or home-sleep apnea test (HSAT).

At minimum, these devices serve to engage patients. Initial clinical questions may inquire about the reason a patient chose to monitor their sleep—What are their sleep concerns? This can easily lead into an open discussion about their sleep as well as the findings from their CST. This leads to a conversation about their expectations regarding their potential sleep disorder, their expectations around their CST and patient-generated health data (PGHD, including clinician review of the data in either a synchronous manner during their clinic visit or asynchronously), and whether or not there will be billing for remote patient monitoring (RPM) of these data. A conversation around data accuracy is essential to set expectations for both parties.

Further, CST can be a powerful way to disseminate information to patients in a self-guided manner. Education surrounding sleep disorders including obstructive sleep apnea (OSA), insomnia, injurious behaviors such as REM sleep behavior disorder (RBD), circadian sleep-wake rhythm disorders (CSWDs), restless legs syndrome (RLS), or disorders of central hypersomnolence can be delivered via short videos or articles available to patients through websites or apps. This may include information about the various disorders as well as guidance for when to seek medical attention.

CST may allow consumers to navigate through their sleep concerns by inputting answers to question prompts and can combine this information with data collected by their wearable or nearable technology, thus leading to a personalized analysis of their sleep concerns and metrics. This collaborative personalization can be further enabled by their sleep clinician, who can assess all of these data and provide vetted educational content and medical expertise.

Sleep concerns, blogs, and sleep-related Google searches increased during the pandemic.[6,7] Americans reportedly Google nearly 5 million sleep queries monthly with sleep apnea, insomnia, and narcolepsy being the most frequent sleep disorder type searches.[8] When determining whether or not to use CST in the care of patients, it is helpful to have an outline of potential use cases, either by symptoms or age/comorbid conditions. One proposed schema is outlined here.

SNORING/OSA SCREENING

Snoring is a very common reason that consumers begin to monitor their sleep. Many apps allow for recording during the sleep period and allow the consumer to both hear and visually see the acoustic signals associated with their snoring. Often, there is a measurement of snoring from mild to heroic, and apneas are often found during these recordings. Several fitness trackers have incorporated oximetry, which also provides information that may encourage consumers to seek further medical attention. Because the vast majority of CSTs are categorized by the FDA as under "wellness" devices/apps, they often contain a disclaimer about medical usage but provide information that helps consumers understand that they may benefit from a formal sleep evaluation. As noted earlier, the use of AI/ML algorithms and added sensors such as pulse oximetry and PPG have moved some CST toward FDA clearance for clinical uses such as apnea screening.

CIRCADIAN RHYTHM DISORDERS INCLUDING JET LAG

These disorders are likely underdiagnosed, and many do not come to medical attention. Patients often are content to consider themselves morning larks or night owls. Google has allowed patients to learn more about their circadian rhythm, and many websites discussing circadian rhythm disorders have emerged with message boards and crowd-sourced information. Fitness tracker data are often shared among community members with advice flowing freely. Many of these patients only seek medical attention when there is a possibility to explore prescription light therapies and/or medications to regulate their circadian rhythm disorder, such as a wake-promoting agent, melatonin, hypnotic, or medication intended to regulate a non–24-hour rhythm. Patients may be well-informed and have collected data for an extended period. These PGHD may shorten the time from initial presentation to final diagnosis by virtue of having access to extended personalized data.

EVALUATION OF HYPERSOMNIAS

Actigraphy has traditionally been used to analyze sleep timing and duration when evaluating complaints of hypersomnia. It is typically used prior to multiple sleep latency testing (MSLT) when exploring the possibility of an organic hypersomnia such as narcolepsy or idiopathic hypersomnia (IH). These devices are expensive, and many clinics, including some at prestigious academic institutes, do not routinely perform actigraphy due to expense and the risk for device loss. Allowing for more robust assessment of our patients, CST may now offer a practical alternative solution to tracking daytime napping and total 24/7 sleep times over extended periods.

INSOMNIA

Sleep concerns and interest in sleep tracking were fueled during the COVID-19 pandemic. Zitting et al. reported a 58% increase in Google searching the word "insomnia" during the first 5 months of 2020 compared with 3 years earlier.[7] Sleep trackers often claim to discern not just sleep from wakefulness but also to provide sleep quality and/or sleep staging information. These data are often displayed in the context of a "sleep score" or will display the percentage of time spent in a given sleep stage. Some CST also provides guidance on establishing an appropriate wind-down routine, proper sleep hygiene measures, light/darkness or naps, and caffeine suggestions, or it may provide personalized lights or sounds for sleep onset and offset. Some devices use headbands to provide acoustic binaural beats and claim to "deepen" sleep. They may provide electroencephalogram (EEG) tracings paired with advice on how to interpret these signals. Some consumers find these to be helpful, while others develop sleep anxiety and orthosomnia (see later).

Intersection: When Consumers Become Patients

As previously noted, fitness trackers are popular with one of five Americans routinely wearing trackers. As these numbers continue to climb, it is inevitable that consumers will begin to notice abnormalities in their sleep, whether this is sleep fragmentation, snoring, or awareness of being sleepier than their cohorts. These consumers may seek medical attention based on these findings. Clinicians, therefore, must be familiar with CST and have an understanding of the CST data accuracy. Although these devices may not replace formal testing at the moment, they may do so in the near future with the addition of more accurate sensors and advanced AI/ML algorithms. At minimum, these devices serve to engage patients, increase their awareness of the importance of sleep, and encourage them to seek further counsel from their primary care or sleep medicine clinicians.

Intersection: Is It Consumer or Medical Grade Technology?

More recently, some CST used complex proprietary AI/ML algorithms derived from multiple sensor data to provide a CST with more advanced data outputs such as sleep stages or AHI. A simple example of a PPG sensor that is added to some wearable CST devices is a pulse oximeter (p/ox). P/ox output is derived from an optical sensor that uses light and a photodetector to create a plethysmography tracing that measures volumetric changes associated with pulsatile arterial blood flow. This signal is affected by the type of light (red, infrared, green), light/detector type (absorption or reflective), sensor location (fingertip, ring, wrist, forehead, earlobe, other), motion artifact, and skin pigmentation to name a few factors. The signal is passed through proprietary AI/ML algorithms that are often derived from a limited population dataset of subjects who may be healthy or may have an array of comorbid medical conditions. Consumer p/oxs may be purchased over the counter and are not intended for medical use, diagnosis, decision making, or treatment. Even medical grade p/oxs have accuracy limitations. For FDA clearance, the current standard is that 66% of p/ox SpO_2 values must be within 2% and 3% of blood gas numbers, and ~95% must be within 4% to 6% of blood gases. In other words, in a well-adult person, a medical grade p/ox with an SpO_2 of 90% may have an acceptable range of 86% to 94%.[9] Adding PPG and accelerometer data (that is enhanced by proprietary "black box" AI/ML algorithms) has provided FDA clearance as an HSAT to a few currently transitioned CST devices.

Orthosomnia

Dr. Kelly Baron was the first to use the term *orthosomnia* when describing patients whose preoccupation with obtaining perfect sleep metrics caused them to develop insomnia.[10] She notes that this phenomenon is important to identify and address as it may further deteriorate their sleep. A brief intervention with cessation of CST device/app utilization and patient education often resolves this issue.

Data Accuracy

Although both consumers and clinicians seek assurance that the CST product claims are accurate for the intended purposes and populations, confirming data accuracy poses several challenges. First, it is not possible for busy clinicians to be familiar with all of the vast number of available sleep CST apps, devices, or their terminologies or data reports. In response, the AASM has provided guides on approaches to evaluating CST apps/devices.[3,11,12] Additional sleep technology educational "Emerging Technology" resources through the AASM and a library of clinical and CST device/app reviews also may be found using the AASM #SleepTechnology resource.[13,14] When attempting to confirm claimed uses, clinicians may find FDA terms confusing and/or may be unable to find validated, peer-reviewed studies to support the specific device/app claim. For example, *FDA registered* simply means that the FDA is aware of the manufacturer and product. *FDA registered* does not mean that it is *FDA cleared* (usually used for Class 2 devices) or *FDA approved* (usually used for Class 3 devices), that the FDA logo may be used, or that the product may be used for medical diagnosis, treatment, or medical decision making.

Data Privacy and Data Access

Clinicians are familiar with research study data being de-identified, not shared outside of the study personnel, and destroyed at the study conclusion. CST allows consumers to self-track sleep and bedroom movements, and CST often allows users to share reports with their clinicians or others. However, most CSTs require the consumer to accept product privacy notices that their sleep and bedroom data are stored on company clouds and may be shared with third business and/or marketing partners. Sharing personal data with businesses presents a potential conflict of interest, and sharing personal data with insurers poses additional medical coverage concerns. Online hackers warrant further data privacy and access concerns, and health care data are reported to be a favorite target for hackers.[15-20]

Financial Considerations

The advantages and disadvantages of monitoring sleep device data, such as CPAP data, are familiar concepts to apnea patients and sleep clinicians. Patient engagement in utilizing CPAP device educational apps and self-monitoring data has been shown to increase therapy compliance, which results in improved clinical outcomes.[21,22] Physician engagement in utilizing these data at visits or between visits may help identify abnormal CPAP data that results in therapy adjustments and/or recognize other changes.[23-25] Although these advantages improve quality care, related physician and sleep staff time for remote data monitoring has been largely unrecognized by insurers to date although there are RPM codes which may prove fruitful. To date, however, the documentation and other requirements are onerous leaving most of this additional work uncompensated since only 25% of practices have used this code, certainly even fewer in the field of sleep medicine.[26] Durable medical equipment (DME) companies balance cost benefits of monitoring the first 90 days of CPAP data to improve CPAP compliance and insurance payments against the costs of added overhead and staff for such data monitoring. Moreover, busy clinicians review CPAP device data and reports generally for two or perhaps three CPAP device manufacturers. This noted, it is not feasible for clinicians, or anyone, to learn to monitor every type of the vast array of CST apps/devices and their reports. An option may be for patients to become familiar with their personal "normal" CST data and data trends and to alert clinicians when they note changes, particularly if accompanied by symptoms.

Liabilities

CSTs are non-prescription devices/apps. Although some CSTs may be considered wellness products promoting improved health and sleep, they generally are not FDA cleared or approved. Few have peer-reviewed publications or evidence supporting claimed uses. Few indicate whether claimed uses are valid across age groups and diverse populations or for healthy patients versus those with sleep or medical conditions. Sleep clinicians thus are hesitant to rely on CST data when forming clinical diagnosis, ordering tests, prescribing treatments, or advising patients.

Some CST provides added medical-grade sensors (e.g., pulse oximetry) but may not have validated the claimed report outputs of the total device or for the intended population. Unless patients are responsible for continuously monitoring their personal data, abnormal data (such as showing hypoxia) could collect without review on a server. If clinicians are provided with an application programming interface (API) for such CST data access, it is of concern that best practices and standards for abnormal CST data alerts and responsibilities are not yet developed or available to clinicians.

Future Considerations

CST use has dramatically increased over the past decade, and the recent COVID-19 pandemic further catalyzed the growth and popularity of consumer interest in self-monitoring of physiological data. This accelerated consumer interest coupled with expanded use of sensors and AI/ML algorithms has further propelled CST to evolve rapidly from its youthful stages. Similar to the transition from childhood through puberty to adulthood, CST devices/apps must continue to develop technically and with imagination, but they also require guard rails such as FDA rules and "best practice" clinical guidelines to ensure safe implementation in medical decision making and clinical care.

As discussed earlier, there are many benefits to consumer use of CST. In particular, if providing accurate sleep-related data, consumers can become patients who are engaged in improving their sleep and self-monitoring their personal sleep and related physiological data. For the provider and staff, monitoring such vast datasets of so many and varied devices/apps is not practical or financially feasible. Providers are further challenged by the rapidly increasing number of CSTs that are hybrid or transitioning medical devices/apps. Such devices may have one output (such as SpO_2) that is FDA cleared but not have other outputs (such as AHI or sleep stages) cleared. For a provider to use the device for diagnosis, treatment, or medical decision making, the device requires FDA clearance or approval of the entire device sensors, advanced and FDA-cleared software as medical device (SaMD) software, and consistent calculated outputs that are to be used clinically.

Some CSTs have claimed data outputs of AHI and sleep staging. The technology is here now for the transition of some devices to provide HSAT-type data outputs for diagnosing apnea. Physiological signals can be collected using PPG and accelerometry for one or for multiple nights. Signals are processed using AI/ML algorithms with the intention of providing HSAT-type data outputs. However, for medical use, the device must demonstrate Class 2 FDA clearance (or Class 3 FDA approval) standards to be used for diagnosis, treatment, or medical decision making. Providers should be aware that many current consumer devices that claim to generate AHI and sleep stages often have disclaimers that these data are not to be used for medical purposes. Providers also should be aware that there appears to be rapid transitioning of some of these consumer devices obtaining FDA clearance/approval as HSAT diagnostic devices.

For consumer use, patients who monitor their personal CST sleep data may alert their provider when device/app data alerts are provided or when there is a change in the pattern of their typical sleep data. Such sleep data might become a self-monitored "vital sign" like heart rate, blood pressure, respiratory rate, or weight. Analysis of large, diverse "sleep vital sign" datasets may provide population health applications for use with comorbid chronic disease management such as for diabetes, cardiovascular disease, or cancer. For example, CST data have been reported to predict pre-symptomatic COVID-19.[27,28]

CSTs are popular and allow massive amounts of individual and group consumer data to be collected over extended periods. If used for medical purposes, the oversight and management of such vast (FDA-cleared device) datasets require validated AI/ML algorithms and alerts. Integration with electronic health records would require frequently scheduled programs to scan such data and to provide appropriate alerts for abnormal data in real time. In a recent randomized prospective study, Yao et al. found an improvement in clinical outcomes for atrial fibrillation patients who participated in a study implementing a mobile health-technology pathway. In addition to other costs, the study protocol required added resources such as training researchers and patients on how to use the app.[29] For a standardized clinical implementation of synchronous and asynchronous monitoring of E-data, reimbursement for added clinical resources as well as best practice guides and models are needed in real-world clinical settings for each CST device/app data type and its proposed use in specified populations.

References

1. Vogels EA. *About One-in-Five Americans Use a Smart Watch or Fitness Tracker.* https://www.pewresearch. org/fact-tank/2020/01/09/about-one-in-five-americans-use-a-smart-watch-or-fitness-tracker/. Accessed March 1, 2024.
2. Stables J. *Wearables Popularity Soars in 2020—and Huawei Is the Big Winner.* https://www.wareable.com/ news/wearables-popularity-soars-in-2020-8322. Accessed March 1, 2024.
3. Khosla S, Deak MC, Gault D, et al. Consumer sleep technology: an American Academy of Sleep Medicine position statement. *J Clin Sleep Med.* 2018;14(5):877-880.
4. Thomas RJ, Bianchi MT. Urgent need to improve PAP management: the devil is in two (fixable) details. *J Clin Sleep Med.* 2017;13(5):657-664.
5. Chinoy ED, Cuellar JA, Huwa KE, et al. Performance of seven consumer sleep-tracking devices compared with polysomnography. *Sleep.* 2021;44(5):zsaa291.
6. *Top 100 Sleep Blogs and Websites.* Feedspot. Available at: https://blog.feedspot.com/sleep_blogs/. Accessed March 1, 2024.
7. Zitting KM, Lammers-van der Holst HM, Yuan RK, et al. Google Trends reveals increases in Internet searches for insomnia during the 2019 coronavirus disease (COVID-19) global pandemic. *J Clin Sleep Med.* 2021;17(2):177-184.
8. Hyde M. *Googling Sleep: What 237 Million Google Searches Reveal About Sleep Problems Across America.* Amerisleep. Available at: https://amerisleep.com/blog/google-searches-and-sleep/. Accessed March 1, 2024.
9. U.S. Food and Drug Administration. *Pulse Oximeter Accuracy and Limitations: FDA Safety Communication.* Available at: https://www.fda.gov/medical-devices/safety-communications/pulse-oximeter-accuracy-and-limitations-fda-safety-communication. Accessed March 1, 2024.
10. Baron KG, Abbott S, Jao N, et al. Orthosomnia: are some patients taking the quantified self too far? *J Clin Sleep Med.* 2017;13(2):351-354.
11. Khosla S, Deak MC, Gault D, et al. Consumer sleep technologies: how to balance the promises of new technology with evidence-based medicine and clinical guidelines. *J Clin Sleep Med.* 2019;15(1):163-165.
12. Schutte-Rodin S, Deak MC, Khosla S, et al. Evaluating consumer and clinical sleep technologies: an American Academy of Sleep Medicine update. *J Clin Sleep Med.* 2021;17(11):2275-2282.
13. *Emerging Technology.* American Academy of Sleep Medicine. Available at: https://aasm.org/clinical-resources/emerging-technology/. Accessed March 1, 2024.
14. *#SleepTechnology.* American Academy of Sleep Medicine. Available at: https://aasm.org/consumer-clinical-sleep-technology/. Accessed March 1, 2024.
15. Davis J. *Top Health IT Security Challenges? Medical Devices, Cloud Security.* Xtelligent Healthcare Media. Available at: https://healthitsecurity.com/news/top-health-it-security-challenges-medical-devices-cloud-security. Accessed March 1, 2024.
16. Davis J. *Healthcare Accounts for 79% of All Reported Breaches, Attacks Rise 45%.* Available at: https:// healthitsecurity.com/news/healthcare-accounts-for-79-of-all-reported-breaches-attacks-rise-45. Accessed March 1, 2024.
17. Ghosh S. *71% of Healthcare Medical Apps Have a Serious Vulnerability; 91% Fail Crypto Tests.* Available at: https://aithority.com/ait-featured-posts/71-of-healthcare-medical-apps-have-a-serious-vulnerability-91-fail-crypto-tests. Accessed March 1, 2024.
18. *Cryptographic Vulnerabilities, Data Leakage and Other Security Breaches in Healthcare Apps.* Security. Available at: https://www.securitymagazine.com/articles/93524-cryptographic-vulnerabilities-data-leakage-and-other-security-breaches-in-healthcare-apps. Accessed March 1, 2024.
19. Horowitz BT. *Mobile Health Apps Leak Sensitive Data Through APIs, Report Finds.* FierceHealthcare. Available at: https://www.fiercehealthcare.com/tech/mobile-health-apps-leak-sensitive-data-through-apis-report-finds. Accessed March 1, 2024.
20. Wetsman N. *Over 40 Million People Had Health Information Leaked This Year: Hacks and Thefts of Health Data Spiked in 2021.* TheVerge-VoxMedia. Available at: https://www.theverge.com/2021/12/8/22822202/ health-data-leaks-hacks. Accessed March 1, 2024.
21. Comstock J. *ResMed's Patient Engagement App Improves PAP Adherence by 17 Percent.* Mobihealth. Available at: https://www.mobihealthnews.com/content/resmeds-patient-engagement-app-improves-pap-adherence-17-percent. Accessed March 1, 2024.

22. Comstock J. *Philips Finds SleepMapper App Boosts CPAP Adherence 22 Percent*. Mobihealth. Available at: https://www.mobihealthnews.com/33742/philips-finds-sleepmapper-app-boosts-cpap-adherence-22-percent. Accessed March 1, 2024.
23. Thomas A, Langley R, Pabary R. Feasibility and efficacy of active remote monitoring of home ventilation in pediatrics. *Pediatr Pulmonol*. 2021;56(12):3975-3982.
24. Tan M, Keenan B, Staley B, et al. Using an Electronic Health Record (EHR) to identify chronic CPAP users with abnormal HL7 CPAP data. *Sleep*. 2018;41(1):402.
25. Pépin JL, Tamisier R, Hwang D, et al. Does remote monitoring change OSA management and CPAP adherence? *Respirology*. 2017;22(8):1508-1517.
26. Leventhal Rajiv Remote patient monitoring use ascends, but most clinicians still aren't adopters. https://www.insiderintelligence.com/content/remote-patient-monitoring-use-ascends-most-clinicians-still-aren-t-adopters, 2023. [Accessed 25 Jan 2024].
27. Mishra T, Wang M, Metwally AA, et al. Pre-symptomatic detection of COVID-19 from smartwatch data. *Nat Biomed Eng*. 2020;4:1208-1220.
28. Quer G, Radin JM, Gadaleta M, et al. Wearable sensor data and self-reported symptoms for COVID-19 detection. *Nat Med*. 2021;27:73-77.
29. Yao Y, Guo Y, Lip GYH, mAF-App II Trial investigators. The effects of implementing a mobile health–technology supported pathway on atrial fibrillation–related adverse events among patients with multi-morbidity: the mAFA-II Randomized Clinical Trial. *JAMA Netw Open*. 2021;4(12):e2140071.

Note: Page numbers followed by *b* indicate boxes *f* indicate figures, and *t* indicate tables.